GONG THERAPY

GONG THERAPY

SOUND HEALING

AND YOGA

MEHTAB BENTON

Bookshelf Press

Gong Therapy: Sound Healing and Yoga
Copyright © 2016 by Michael Benton

All rights reserved. No part of this book may be used or reproduced by any means, graphic, electronic, or mechanical, including photocopying, recording, taping or by any information storage system without the written permission of the publisher except in the case of brief quotations embodied in critical articles and reviews.

Foreign publication rights available from the publisher.

Bookshelf Press books may be ordered by contacting:

Bookshelf Press
PO Box 50028
Austin, TX 78763
www.bookshelfpress.com
orders@bookshelfpress.com

You should not undertake any exercise or therapeutic regimen recommended in this book before consulting your personal physician. Neither the author nor the publisher shall be responsible or liable for any loss or damage allegedly arising as a consequence of your use or application of any information or suggestions contained in this book.

Cover and interior art by Logynn Lyons

ISBN: 978-1-939239-11-2 (hc)

Library of Congress Control Number: 2016909440
Printed in the United States of America

The Gong has the power of creativity.

Absolutely it is a therapy.

And it can expand the mind

beyond its horizon.

Yogi Bhajan

Contents

Introduction 1

Healing, Yoga and Sound 5
    Yoga and the Gong
    Healing and the Sound of the Gong
    Physical Healing
    Emotional Healing
    Spiritual Healing
    The Gong Player as Therapist

The Structure of a Gong Therapy Session 15
    Client Education
    Client Evaluation and Assessment
    Selection of Methodology
    Preparing the Gong Therapy Environment
        Positioning the Client
        Positioning the Gongs
    Gong Playing Session
    Client Integration
    Closure and Follow-Up

Gong Therapy Methodology 31
    Asanas: Body Positions of Gong Therapy
    Drishtis: Role of the Eyes in Gong Therapy
    Mudras: Hand Positions in Gong Therapy
        Mudras for Symptoms and Disease
        Mudras for Chakras, Elements and Doshas
    Pranayama: Role of the Breath in Gong Therapy
    Mantras: Affirmations and Sacred Sounds
    Yoga Nidra: Relaxation and Guided Meditation
        Guided Relaxation and Visualization for the Chakras
        Healing Light Yoga Nidra
        Point-to-Point Deep Relaxation

Gongs for Therapy 91
    Selecting the Gong Stand
    Selecting the Mallets
    Therapeutic Gongs

Gong Playing Techniques for Therapy   101
　　　Three Basic Components of Gong Playing
　　　　　Gong Playing Areas
　　　　　Rhythm and Volume in Therapeutic Playing
　　　Patterns and Contrasts: The Essence of Playing the Gong
　　　　　Therapeutic Playing Patterns
　　　　　Two Healing Polarities: Langhana and Brimhana

Group Gong Therapy   127
　　　Group Assessment
　　　Group Therapy Environment
　　　Group Therapy Methodology
　　　Group Therapy Yoga Classes
　　　　　Releasing Fears
　　　　　Nervous System Regeneration

Gong Therapy as a Profession   135

Gong is the only instrument that can create the vibration of affirmativity. Life become yes to you and the word no is eliminated from your dictionary

Yogi Bhajan

Introduction

Gong Therapy began before the first gong in the world was ever struck by its maker. The act of creating a gong was a transformational process in itself, changing forever its creator and all those who heard it.

How could it be otherwise? The sound of the Gong opens the portal to another realm of consciousness and, as such, is a sacred instrument that sanctifies those around it.

It reminds us of the universe, before it came into form, and of the nature of the soul, before it became embodied in the limitations of time and space. Its cosmic resonance does what all therapy is made to do – reminds us of who we truly are and not what we think we have become.

So whenever the Gong is played, therapy occurs because transformation occurs, and we have a new relationship to the body, mind and spirit that invites healing to occur.

In my other books, *Gong Yoga: Healing and Transformation through Sound* and *Teaching Gong Yoga: Theory and Practice*, I have detailed the special relationship the gong has with sound, healing and spiritual practices. This book is about applying the sound of the gong as a one-on-one healing modality for therapists, teachers, and healers who want to engage clients in a personalized journey to wellness that goes beyond the usual experience most people have with the gong in yoga classes and group relaxation sessions.

As such, there is an emphasis in this book on the individual and how to create a gong session that addresses specific needs and desired outcomes, and that also takes into account a person's health history and current challenges, so that specific methodologies may be used effectively with the sound healing.

Gong Therapy also assumes that there may need to be multiple sessions to fully complete the healing journey of the individual, and that there may be an on-going counseling and therapeutic relationship between the gong player and the client.

For this reason, Gong Therapy is best practiced by healthcare professionals and by those who understand the unique nature of a client-healer relationship. If you have a background in other therapeutic or counseling professions, this book can help you apply the techniques of the gong and sound healing with your clients. If your only experience with the gong before this book has been playing for groups, classes and in relaxation sessions, then you will need to proceed slowly as you enter the role of a therapist as this book does not purport to make you one by simply following the instructions within.

With this disclaimer, this book can help you play the gong in a way that will help many people as they take responsibility for their healing journey. You will be able to create a space where self-healing can occur more easily, and you can facilitate experiences that can be empowering and life-changing for your clients.

Other than the technical ability and experience to play the gong, the other requirement for a gong therapist is a sustained daily meditative practice and a willingness to set the individual ego aside in service to the person who is in front of you. Remember that the gong itself is the healing instrument, yet it is your pure intention and alignment with the divine will that directs its healing.

As with my other books on the Gong, this book is greatly indebted to my spiritual teacher, Yogi Bhajan the master of Kundalini Yoga and the Gong, and is founded squarely on the principles and practices of yoga.

While Gong Therapy exists in other forms and formats independent of yoga, my choice is to embrace this path because it provides a proven and safe container for the changes that Gong Therapy can create in both the practitioner and the client.

If you are drawn to these words, if you have felt the power and majesty of the gong, and if you desire to help others attain their optimal expression of health and Self, then welcome to this emerging discipline of therapeutic sound healing that will transform the lives of all the people you touch.

Physical sound can lead you to the

Inner vibrations of prana.

Prana is the cause of all sound,

And sound is the expression of prana.

Swami Satchidananda

Healing, Yoga and Sound

To understand the principles and practices of Gong Therapy, we must first understand the relationship between sound and healing.

Healing can be defined as the restoration of the natural balance and flow of energy on all levels of existence: physical, mental, emotional and spiritual. This definition asserts that health is the natural state of an organism, and illness or disease occurs when this state is deranged by an imbalance or lack of vital life force energy.

In the practice of Yoga, this vital energy is called *prana*. Prana is the propulsive force that causes all things to come into existence, to breathe, to live, and ultimately to change and disappear through time. In yoga, it is said that prana is the link between matter and energy, between nature and consciousness, and the bridge to self-realization.

All of yoga, in whatever form it is practiced, is based upon the cultivation, consolidation and circulation of prana. It is through prana that consciousness is changed, and it is the presence of prana in the body that insures health and well-being.

All healing is predicated on the availability and movement of prana through the physical body. Prana comes from food, air, water, light, and ultimately sound.

For example, prana is transferred through the element of earth and the sense of smell by the food we eat. Some foods, such as leafy greens, are high in prana while other foods, such as decaying meat, are low in prana.

Prana is transferred through the element of water and the sense of taste by the fluids we drink. Some fluids are high in prana, such as mountain streams, while others are low, such as stagnant water.

Prana comes to us through the element of fire and the sense of sight through light and heat, such as the prana present in sunlight. Environments full of light, such as deserts, are high in prana while areas low in natural light, such as confined spaces, are low in prana.

Prana is transferred through the element of air and the sense of touch, through the air we breathe and the feel of wind on the skin.

Again, environments that are airy and invite circulation are high in prana while locations with poor air quality are low in prana.

Finally, prana is transferred through the element of space, or ether, and assimilated through the sense of hearing. Sounds that are expansive and move harmoniously through space are higher in prana than sounds that are discordant, damped or muffled.

In the same way the five elements move from the grossest (earth) to the subtlest (space), so does prana become more refined as we move from the fundamental sense of smell to the developed sense of hearing, and similarly from the grossest carrier of prana, food, to the subtlest carrier of prana, sound.

Sound carried through the element of ether and perceived by the sense of hearing, as well as celestial sound that transcends the physical senses, is the most ethereal and subtle agent of prana, and is the most effective healing agent for the energy body.

This relationship between the sound of the gong, healing, and the energy body exists, because all sound is essentially the expression of prana, the vital energy of the universe. The primal sound in yoga, the sound of OM, is said to be the highest level of sound vibration that created time, space, and form. In essence, we are sonic creatures living in a universe created by sound. In sound we are born and in sound we are healed.

Yoga and the Gong

While the Gong can initiate and support healing independently of any accompanying modalities, it is most effective when used with the practices of Yoga, the original holistic healing system. This is especially so when used with the therapeutic branch of yoga, the ancient science of Ayurveda.

Yoga and Ayurveda are based upon perfecting the relationship between the human being and the energy of prana. Both of these Vedic sciences are influenced by the energy of sound healing through the use of mantra and the attunement to the inner sounds heard in the meditative state.

The Gong has been used for hundreds of years in the practice of yoga and meditation, and more recently in the practice of Kundalini Yoga, to accelerate the therapeutic transformation of the yogic practices.

As such, the effectiveness of the gong when used therapeutically is exponentially multiplied when used with the yogic techniques of asanas (postures), pranayama (breath), mantra (sacred sound), and meditation (with relaxation).

While Gong therapy can be practiced without any knowledge or experience of yoga, a Gong therapist is a better therapist if they understand the relationship that exists between yoga and the gong.

Healing and the Sound of the Gong

In the same manner that sound is the source of all prana, one can assert that the Gong is the mother of all sound. As Yogi Bhajan, the master of the Gong and Kundalini Yoga, said: "The gong is not a musical instrument; the gong is God. It is the most pure sound that man could create, out of which come all music, all sounds, and all words."

The gong works on all levels to heal and transform. From the purely physical, to the emotional and spiritual, the sound of the gong can promote a positive change in the listener. In addition to yogis and yoga teachers, doctors, music therapists, psychotherapists, and researchers have used the gong as an adjunct to their healing modalities.

Physical Healing

The sound of the gong has proven to be effective in addressing many symptoms that accompany physical illnesses and diseases, from providing pain relief to aiding in regeneration. For example, the condition of tinnitus (continual ringing in the ears) responds very well to the gong, especially when it is played strongly. Most people report immediate and short-term relief for up to several days, and in some cases for a much longer period or even a complete healing of the condition. Similarly, the symptoms of vertigo (dizziness) also lessen after listening to the gong. Headaches often disappear after a gong session, and several people have reported that misalignments in the spine are removed after they have experienced the gong.

These healing episodes result when the person hears the gong played live, not in a recorded manner, because the sound waves transfer the living energy of the player in the moment that the gong is played. One theory about the healing quality of the gong being played live is that it produces a strong sound wave, almost tangible to the touch, which stimulates the physical body by influencing the surface of the skin. The sonic touch of the gong can be a healing touch as its sound stimulates the body's dermatomes.

Dermatomes are surface areas of skin extending from the spine throughout the body. Through a network of nerves, these skin areas are connected to different organs in the body and with corresponding segments of the spinal cord. These skin areas can be stimulated by sound waves, much like a massage, and produce effects on corresponding organs and other areas of the body.

The gong is especially effective in stimulating the dermatomes when played in a reasonable proximity to the listener, as is the case during a private gong therapy session. Particularly when the gong is played within three feet (one meter) of the listener, a low frequency sound wave is created that can encase the body in a sonic envelope akin to a continuous massage.

Educator and musician Johannes Heimrath conducted many workshops and healing sessions with the gong through the 1980s in Germany. He discovered that the sound of the gong was most helpful in relieving neck pain and headaches, menstrual difficulties and cramping in the chest and upper respiratory system.

Anne Kathrin Nickel and her associate researchers published an article in *Music Therapy Today* (September 2003) that also confirmed that the gong, and other instruments, proved helpful in treating children with migraine headaches.

The *European Spine Journal* revealed that the gong was helpful in accelerating the healing process of acute ankle sprains. Anecdotally, a gong player and counselor obtained relief from his sprained ankle by propping his foot directly in front of a 28-inch gong and playing it for 10-15 minutes over several days. In England, a veterinarian plays the gong for horses as part of their sprain treatments to achieve accelerated healing.

On a purely physical level, the sound of a live gong stimulates circulation, while its wide range of frequencies stimulates nerve endings. This may be useful in recovering from injuries in which nerve damage has occurred or from trauma or drug use which have compromised the nervous system. The sound of the gong stimulates the glandular system to a higher level of functioning, and in particular the pituitary and pineal glands seem directly affected by its sound.

Finally, as physical distress and illness often have an emotional and stress-related component, the gong affects the physical health by working in these areas as well.

Emotional Healing

As the sound of the gong creates deep relaxation, clears the mind, and stimulates the glandular system to a higher level of functioning, it also aids in the reorganization of the emotional energy and feelings that are tied into the body structure and consequently affect the mind.

In his book *Music and Healing Across Cultures* (2006), musical therapist David Akombo shared his research on the use of the Gamelan Gong as a historical way that schizophrenia has been treated in the Balinese culture. The illness is often viewed as much as a spiritual illness as a physical illness in Southeastern Asian society and the gong holds a cultural position as both a physical and spiritual agent in effecting a cure. It is used specifically in the psychiatric hospital to help with the patient's schizophrenia.

In 1999 a study published by the German Society for Music Therapy entitled *"Music Therapy with Archaic Instruments: An Innovative Method for Treating Early Disorders,"* Dr. Peter Hess, neurologist and psychiatrist and director of the Day Clinic Metznerpark, Frankenthal in Germany concluded that the sound of the gong was an effective therapeutic approach for working with psychotic patients. In brief, his research revealed that the trance-like state, or altered state of consciousness, induced by hearing the gong "reveals early biographical layers of consciousness and transpersonal dimensions. The similarity of the experiences in the sound trance and in the psychotic episode gives the patients the chance to integrate them. So a healing process is initiated and the patients' sense of responsibility and independence is supported."

Dorita S. Berger in her book *Music Therapy, Sensory Integration and the Autistic Child* (2002), recounts that no musical instrument seemed to have an effect on her four-year old autistic patient until he heard the gong. In their book *Clinical Applications of Music Therapy in Psychiatry* (1999), therapists Tony Wigram and Jos De Backer give both a recommendation and caveat to using the gong: "The discovery of the gong was a boom to music therapy. The application of the gong became the state of the art. However, many used the gong without any expertise and this holds a danger."

The cautionary perspective on using the gong for healing and therapy is a good one. The gong is a powerful and transformational instrument. Its sound can both heal and destroy. Indeed, it was used in ancient times as both a weapon to disorient enemies as well as an inspiring call to duty. It is akin to a high-speed dentist drill, able to clean out decay or create torturous pain. Simply striking the gong during a healing session, or using it as a therapeutic addendum, may not work and may harm. It is an instrument to respect and use with understanding.

Spiritual Healing

Perhaps the most common symptoms of spiritual malaise today are substance abuse and addictive behavior. Many researchers and therapists have recognized this connection between abusive addictions and spiritual disconnection, including psychiatrist Dr. Ray Matthew, director of the Duke University Addictions Program. His research has shown that the same pleasure centers in the brain stimulated by drugs like marijuana are also activated by spiritual experiences. Matthew observed that the key to breaking the destructive addictive response is to first "detach yourself from the pressure and content of your mind for a minute or two and you become freer from committing compulsive, automatic actions."

The gong is a singularly effective instrument to help the listener detach from the pressure and content of the mind, through an induced meditative state, in order to get free of habitual patterns. The spiritual healing of the gong occurs through the connection it makes between the listener and the world beyond the body and mind. It provides that experience of a non-ordinary and elevating reality that the addict often seeks through drugs.

In one incident, related to me by a San Antonio pediatrician who uses the gong with her young patients, a youngster began to develop a smoking habit, yet no longer had the impulse to smoke after just one gong therapy session with her.

For a number of years, the gong has been used in programs for recovering drug addicts to rebuild the nervous system and to open a spiritual connection. As early as 1973, Yogi Bhajan and his students began a program in Tucson, Arizona called Superhealth that incorporated Kundalini yoga technology and extended gong sessions to treat recovering drug addicts. The program was accredited by the Joint Commission on Accreditation of Healthcare Organization and received its highest commendation. In its first year of operation, it distinguished itself as being in the top 10% of all treatment programs throughout the U.S, with an astounding recovery rate of 91%.

The spiritual healing power of the gong is perhaps best understood by its ability to create a non-ordinary state of transcendent reality and a connection with a vastness beyond the finite self. In this space, even for the briefest of moments, the gong is a portal to what has always existed and what can always be.

The Gong Player as Therapist

The successful practice of Gong Therapy requires that the therapist be both skilled in playing the gong and in facilitating the journey of healing transformation for the client.

In much the same way that the massage therapist uses their hands or the psychotherapist uses their words, the gong therapist uses their gong as their instrumentality for healing and transformation. As such, the Gong therapist needs not only a fundamental technical knowledge of how to play the gong skillfully, but also an appreciation for subtle differences required for playing the gong therapeutically. Without expert training and playing experience, a gong that is played poorly and discordantly can be disruptive to the nervous system and harmful to the listener.

There is far more than technical proficiency, however, required for a gong therapist. Beyond the actual playing instrument and the sound it creates, the ultimate success of a gong therapist requires a developed sense of intuition and sensitivity that comes from a regular spiritual practice (sadhana) in which the ego is managed by the discerning intelligence of the meditative mind.

In addition, the therapist needs the experience, or the natural ability, to form a healthy impersonal relationship with a client based on trust, concern, and a studied neutrality, independent of any personal needs or agenda or desire to impress or even to heal the client. Ultimately, the therapist must see himself or herself as an agent of healing, and not as a healer, to avoid the mistakes made by the self-limiting ego. For this reason, playing the gong as therapy is best done as an act of meditation and service with the intention to awaken the inner healer within the client.

A person does not hear sound

Only through the ears;

He hears sound through

Every pore of the body.

It permeates the entire being,

And according to its particular influence,

Either slows or quickens

The rhythm of the blood circulation;

It either awakens or soothes

The nervous system.

Hazrat Inayat Khan

Structure of a Gong Therapy Session

In many ways, the structure of a gong therapy session follows the same guidelines and sequence for most client-centered therapeutic work, regardless of modality.

The sequence consists of these phases:

- Client Education
- Client Evaluation and Assessment
- Selection of Methodology
- Preparation of Environment
- Gong Playing Session
- Client Integration
- Closure and Follow-Up

Depending upon the client's needs and the therapist skills, the entire session can be done in a single meeting that lasts from 30 to 90 minutes. Some therapists prefer to do the initial education and assessment in a separate preliminary meeting in order to prepare for the therapy session.

Client Education

The first job of the therapist is to educate the client about the therapeutic process, answer questions, and set expectations.

You may wish to show them where the therapy session will be conducted and how they will be positioned. You may want to introduce them to the gongs, what types they are, how you will use them, and even allow them to hear how they sound (especially if they have never heard a gong played before).

Explain how the sound, while it may seem loud or close, is not harmful to the hearing in anyway at the level and for the length of time they are played. If they have heard the gong before but never have had the experience of being so close to them as when they are being used in therapy, they may feel the sound more intensely in their body and let them now that this is part of the healing process.

Remind them that the most important thing is to simply relax and let the gongs do the work. Explain how the sound of the gong is unique in its ability to transform and how it has been used throughout time to create a new relationship to the body, mind and spirit.

Share with the client your experience in working with the gongs, the results your clients have received, and the importance for them to set an intention for their session.

Let them understand that part of the therapeutic process is to release of old patterns, and that as thoughts or feelings arise, simply let them go with the sound of the gong, much like the cleansing waves of the ocean.

Allow them to ask questions or express concerns and then take the time to actively listen rather than preemptively explaining everything to them.

Client Evaluation and Assessment

In order to determine the methodology and playing techniques to use during the gong therapy session, the therapist needs to evaluate the client's current condition and experience with the gong and sound healing to assess the primary reasons and needs of the client for the session.

A verbal interview or a written intake form may include the following questions:

- What is your primary reason for having a gong therapy session?

- How would you describe your current state of physical health? What recurring physical symptoms or recent illnesses have you experienced?

- How would you describe your current state of mental health and emotional well-being?

- Do you have any physical conditions that prevent you from relaxing on your back?

- Do you wear hearing aid devices? Have you experienced any past traumas connected with loud sounds? (If so, they should remove hearing aid devices and given permission to cover the ears with a blanket or use ear plugs during the session if they are sound sensitive.)

- Have you experienced relaxing or listening to the gong before? If so, how many times? Have you ever had any type of sound healing session?

- Do you practice yoga regularly or in the past?

- What would you like to accomplish in your gong therapy session?

- Do you have any questions about the gong or your therapy session?

For first-time clients, these questions may be sufficient for an initial evaluation to plan their gong therapy session.

The therapist may, however, use more sophisticated and thorough evaluation techniques to design follow-up sessions with their clients. For example, you may want to assess which chakras may need attention or which elements or Ayurvedic constitutions (*doshas*) may need balancing.

If you are trained in other therapeutic modalities, such as chiropractic, acupuncture, massage therapy, yoga therapy, Ayurvedic healing, Reiki or other energy and healing work, then you use the knowledge from those approaches to better assess your client's needs.

Selection of Methodology

Based upon the answers from your interview and the client's health history and their reasons for having a gong therapy session, you are now ready to select the various methods and techniques to support their healing process. You will also be able to determine the general playing techniques you will use, as well as the gongs you select and how to use them in the session.

The specific gong therapy methodologies and techniques that can be used in a session are described in the next chapter.

Briefly, they fall into these categories (with the corresponding yoga techniques):

- Body position of the client (Asanas)
- Eye position of the client (Drishtis)
- Hand positions of the client (Mudras)
- Breathing suggestions for the client (Pranayama)
- Affirmations and healing sounds (Mantra)
- Guided relaxation and visualizations (Meditation)

In general, you would use only one technique from a category, and would likely not use techniques from more than three categories, unless the client has had substantial experience with yoga or sound healing. The first session should be kept simple to avoid overburdening the client with too many techniques.

Preparing the Gong Therapy Environment

The gong therapy environment ideally should have a minimum of ambient noise and visual stimulation. The therapy space must be able to accommodate the client either relaxing on the floor or on a massage table while allowing enough room for the gong therapist to position the gong or gongs at the feet of the client, at the head of the client and to either side of the client. At a minimum there should be at least three feet (one meter) space on all sides of the client.

The treatment room or therapy space therefore needs to be approximately 9 feet (3 meters) by 12 feet (4 meters) at a minimum. If more gongs are used, or moved during the treatment session, then space must be allowed for that as well.

If larger gongs (34 inches or greater) are used during the session, then a larger space is needed.

Positioning the Client

The client will typically be lying either on the floor or on a treatment table, such as a standard massage table, which places them about the waist-height of the therapist.

If the client is on the floor, there should be sufficient padding and support to be comfortable for relaxing. Ideally there is 2 to 4 inches (5 to 10 centimeters) of supporting blankets or a small mattress that is covered by a wool pad or other natural fibers. There may be a thin cushion to support the neck if needed.

The primary advantage for the client to be positioned on the floor is that it can allow them to use a restorative yoga position for the session and allow for more movement, if needed, during the session. If a floor stand gong is used, then the gong can be placed near the client. Depending if the floor is wood or non-carpeted, having the client on the floor may also allow the vibrations of the gong to travel along the floor and more closely connect the client to the sound energy.

The disadvantage with having the client on the floor is that the gong player must remain seated to play the gong and limits their movement during the session.

Many therapists find that using a massage or treatment table for the client allows for more efficient positioning of the gongs as well as movement of the gongs should that be necessary during the session. The therapist can also stand, kneel or sit when playing the gong according to their preference.

Positioning the Gongs

For gong therapy sessions, the gongs are placed much closer to the client than is experienced during a yoga class or typical relaxation. The gongs are usually positioned 18 to 36 inches (.5 to 1 meter) from the client's body, depending upon the size of the gong, and where the gong is positioned relative to the client's body.

Ideally the gongs are almost equal in height to the client's body. If the client is on the floor, then the gong is best placed on the floor so the bottom of the gong is not more than 36 inches (1 meter) above the client. If the client is on a treatment table or similar elevated position, then the top of the gong should not be below the client's body.

The near proximity of the gongs creates a powerful experience for the client as the sound waves begin to effect change on a physical level in addition to the subtle healing that also occurs. When the sound of the gong is "felt" along the skin and within the physical body, there is a closer relationship between the sound and the client that allows for a deeper absorption.

The backs of the gongs always face the client when they are used in the close proximity of a gong therapy session. The gong therapist plays the front of the gongs, as is normal, and can maintain visual contact with the client.

The gongs can be placed at the feet of the client, at the head of the client, on the right side of the client, or the left side of the client. All four positions have their uses and advantages.

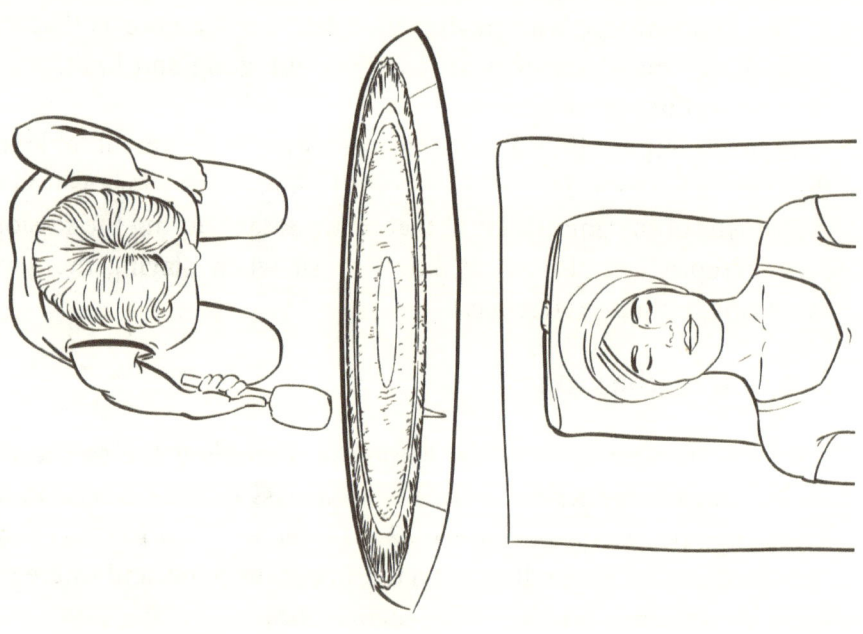

Gongs at the Feet of the Client – This is the most common placement for a gong therapy session. When playing the gong at the feet of the client, the gong can be placed closer to the client's body than in other positions. Clients will generally be more receptive and feel a heightened security when the gong is played at the feet. If multiple positions of the gong are used during the session, beginning at the feet is an excellent starting position as it grounds and stabilizes the client. This is also a good position to end the session if multiple positions or gongs are used.

Playing at the feet of the client also allows energy to move upward through the chakras from the base to the crown. It is helpful for clients who are disconnected from their body, have difficult focusing or being present, as well as psychological and physical conditions connected to the first three chakras.

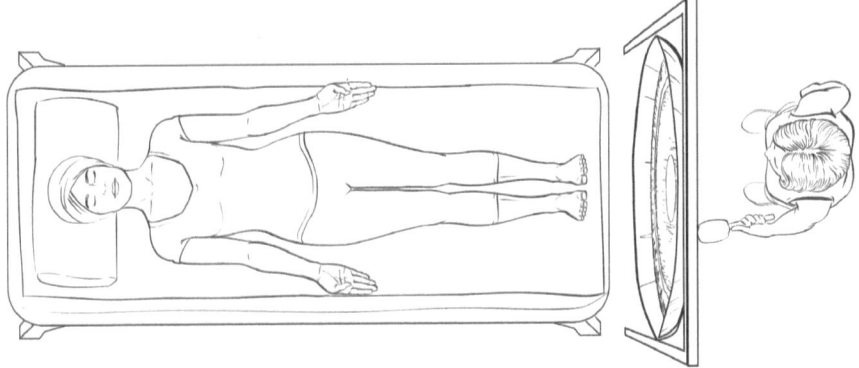

Gongs at the Head of the Client – This is a powerful placement for the gong and has several benefits as well as cautionary considerations. In this position, the gong is farther from the client than in the other positions. The top of the head is extremely sensitive to the gong as its sound activates the crown chakra, and so the gong is also played at a lower volume than in the other positions. If the gong is too close to the head or if the therapist plays too loudly, it can create anxiety and fear as well as mistrust by the client.

Playing at the head of the client does create a deep opening of the self to the infinite. It can serve as a bridge to take the client out of their limited sense of identity and connect them to a deeper understanding of their place in the cosmos. It may prove useful for working with addictions and eating disorders, as well schizophrenia, bipolar episodes, depression and conditions connected to the upper three chakras.

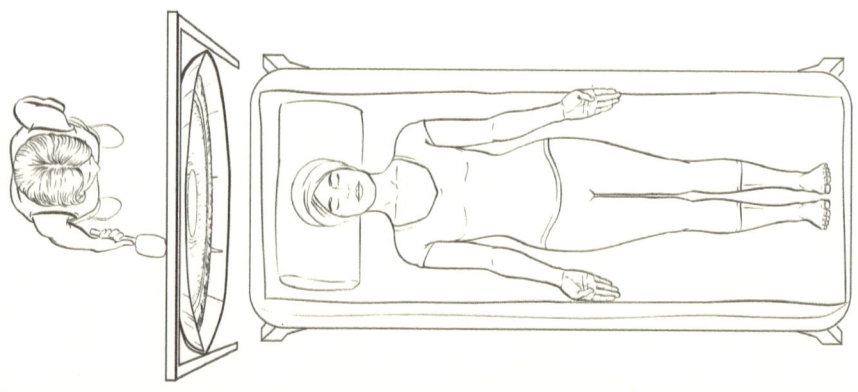

Gongs at the Sides of the Client – These are good secondary positions to create a sense of surrounding sound and enveloping energy when the gong is also played at the feet and/or head of the client. Gongs played on the sides may be positioned almost as close to the client as when played at the feet, provided they are placed below the client's shoulder level.

When gongs are played alternately on both the right and left side of the client, there is a strong balancing of polarities and integration of brain function. Blocks are removed so there is a better flow of energy through the meridians and organs of the body.

When the gong is played only on the **right side** of the client, there is an activation of the **left hemisphere** of the brain, which can be helpful in elevating the mood, activating energy, enhancing the analytic function of the mind, increasing the projective nature of the individual, relieving depression, and healing conditions connected to the male polarity of the individual.

When the gong is played only on the **left side** of the client, there is an activation of the **right hemisphere** of the brain, which can be helpful in creating relaxation, release from tension and anxiety, lowering fear, awakening intuition, and healing conditions connected to the female polarity of the individual.

If multiple gongs and are used in the session, or if the gong is on an easily movable stand, then several gong positions can be used effectively during the session.

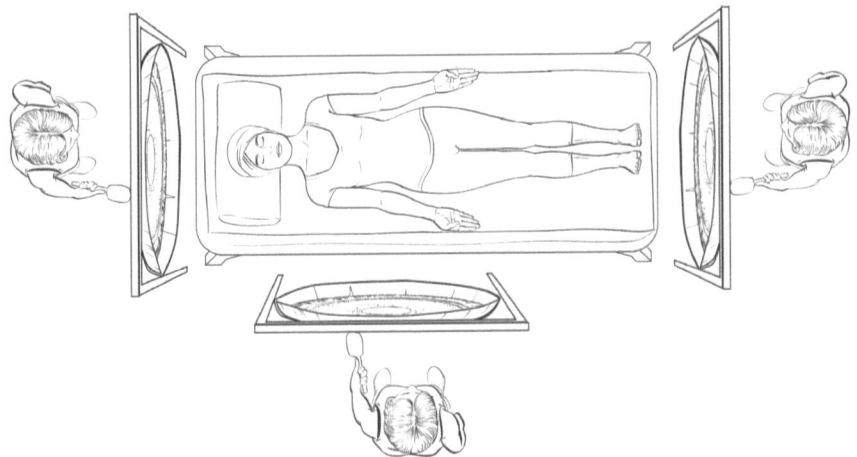

Moving the Gong Around the Client – There are occasions where the gong can be moved around the client while still being played. These is either done by having the gong on a stand with rolling wheels or by using a hand-held gong. If a hand-held gong is used, or if a stand with rolling wheels is high enough, then the gong can be moved directly over the client's body, rather than being at the top, bottom or sides. This is a powerful experience and will move energy quickly.

This technique must be done carefully and skillfully; otherwise it can create anxiety and disorientation in the client. Special care must be exercised when moving the gong around the head. Ideally the gong does not go above the level of the heart and never moves close to the top or side of the head while it is in motion. The gong should also be moved slowly so the client has a sense of the gong's location and orientation and is not startled by the gong suddenly appearing to be in motion.

When done correctly, the sound of a moving gong can create a sense of expansion and openness and an invitation to release into the movement of energy. As this is an advanced technique, it is best used with clients who have already experienced the benefits of gong therapy.

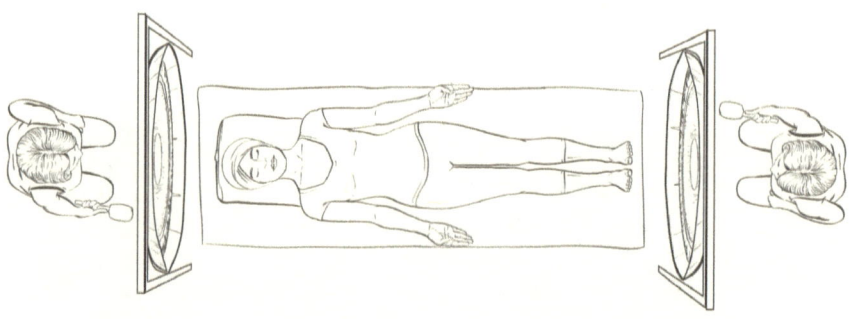

Multiple Positions and Multiple Gongs

Changing the position of the gong during a therapy session, while not always necessary, can be effective in moving blocked energy and accessing different energy centers (chakras) and areas of the physical body. The important consideration is that the changing of positions is not disruptive to the healing process or distracting to the client.

If multiple gongs and stands are available, once the client is in place then the gongs can be positioned for easy access during playing. Ideally the gongs may be on rolling stands so they can easily be positioned or moved during the session. Some stands hold two gongs and this is preferable to moving the gongs from one stand to another.

Multiple gongs can allow for expanding the opportunities during the playing (see "Selecting Gongs for Therapy") and provide a wide range of healing possibilities. Having one or two gongs on moveable stands with wheels also allows for changing position more easily as well.

While a single gong used in only one position can give remarkable results, and may be the only instrument you need, the ability to have two, three or even up to eight gongs used during a session can allow you to refine your practice in highly imaginative ways. However, please proceed slowly with incorporating a lot of gongs and moving them around when you begin your journey as a gong therapist. One gong played well is far better than six gongs played poorly.

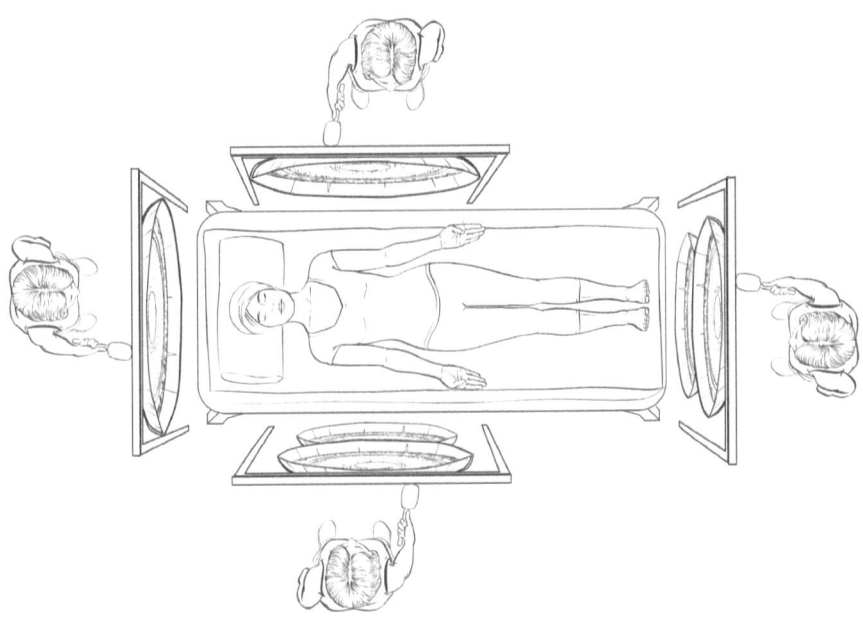

If you work with multiple gong players or therapists, it can be very transformational for several therapists to play the gongs for the client. Obviously this requires a high level of skill and well as intuitive alignment between the therapists.

Gong Playing Session

At the beginning of the session, the therapist gives the client instructions on how to use the various techniques (if any) during the session, such as hand positions, affirmations, and so on. The therapist then allows the client to connect to their breath and begin to relax.

One method for inducing a receptive state for the sound of the gong is to instruct the client to first become aware of the rise and fall of the diaphragm with the breath. Then have the client inhale the breath up from the bottom of the feet to the top of the head and then exhale down from the head to the feet. After several conscious breaths, they can allow the breath to relax and become aware of any sounds around them or any sounds within themselves, such as the sound of their breath or heartbeat.

After a few moments of silence during which the therapist sets intentions, perhaps offering a prayer or a blessing, or using a silent or spoken mantra, the gong is struck once softly. The initial sound is allowed to grow and then slowly fade into a few moments of silence.

If there is more than one gong, it is usually recommended that the playing session begin by first playing the gong at the feet of the client.

The gong is played for a period of 11 to 31 minutes, depending upon the length of the therapy session, and suggestions for playing are given in the chapter, "Gong Playing Techniques for Therapy."

The session may be devoted entirely to working with one specific condition, illness or need, or it can be divided into two or more sections, with pauses to allow for integration, as well as perhaps a change of the modality being used, or to introduce other gongs or playing techniques for the following healing segment.

At the end of the playing session, allow for one to three minutes of silence to prepare the client for a gradual transition to a seated posture for integration.

Client Integration

After the client is guided to a seated position, allow suitable time for integration and grounding, as well as respecting the changes that may have taken place during the session.

If the client chooses to end the silence with a comment, simply acknowledge by re-phrasing their comment into a neutral question to invite additional feedback and processing. For example, if the client says, "That was very interesting." The therapist could respond,

"So it was an interesting experience for you?" or "In what way was it interesting?"

Your role is to allow the client to process their experience by speaking with you without trying to shape their experience. Do not try to explain what happened, or how it happened, or what you did.

These following guidelines may be helpful as you allow the client to integrate their transformational experience:

- Use your language to facilitate the client's own exploration of themselves and simply provide a non-judgmental space in which they can explore their own experience of the session: physical, emotional, and spiritual.

- Instead of engaging them in conversation or analysis, simply repeat back to the client the information they have given you to confirm their own process.

- Do not diagnose the issues or problems with the idea of coming to a conclusion for them. Although you may be able to see their situation from a wider perspective, allow them to make these discoveries and connections for themselves.

- Do not psychoanalyze in any way. Let the client draw conclusions, see relationships and patterns and make a plan of action.

- Re-assure them that whatever may have arisen during the session is natural part of the clearing and healing process.

- Confirm they feel positive about their experience.

You should allow at least 5 to 10 minutes for integration after the session before the client leaves.

Closure and Follow-Up

Before the client leaves, give them suggestions for continuing their healing experience and transformation. If they used mudras, mantras, affirmations, yoga postures or other modalities during the therapy session, let them know they can continue using them at home over the next several days or weeks.

Mudras and mantras are especially easy to do to reconnect afterwards to the gong therapy experience. If you have other healing experience or techniques that may support them (massage, acupuncture, meditation, etc.) please offer those as well.

If possible, see if they wish to schedule a follow-up gong therapy session or perhaps a series of sessions. This is the best time to have them commit to a continuing relationship with you as more than one session may be required to complete their healing process, especially as other issues may arise during their healing journey.

On the day after the gong therapy session, schedule a follow-up communication with them (email, phone call, etc.) to see if other things have come up for them after the session that may be helpful to talk about.

Remember that for many people, a gong therapy session can be deeply transformational and it is useful to remind yourself and the client that the changes often continue beyond the session.

The gong is a brotherhood of tones

Perfectly united and blended, a cosmic entity.

In it the law of cohesion manifests fully.

It is a mass of atoms and molecules:

It is a host of tones, of cosmic lives.

It is a concentric and organic body,

Through which the energy of sound

Flows uninterrupted.

Dane Rudhyar

Gong Therapy Methodology

Gong Therapy combines the sound of the Gong with the methodologies of Yoga to energize and facilitate the movement of energy (*prana*) to heal the body, clear the mind and elevate the consciousness.

The various methods that are used in Gong Therapy include the body position of the client during the therapy session (*asana*), hand positions held during the therapy (*mudras*), breath awareness (*pranayama*), directed internal gazes of the eyes (*drishtis*), affirmations with other sacred sounds (*mantras*), as well as guided visualization and relaxation (*yoga nidra*).

Following the interview and assessment portion of the therapy session, the gong therapist determines which methodologies the client should employ during the playing of the gong. The selection of the methods is influenced by the major conditions to be addressed, as well as the ability and willingness of the client to use these methods.

In some cases, only one method may be used during the session. Indeed, care must be taken not to overwhelm the client by suggesting too many different methods, or changing the methods used during the session. Remember that the methodologies are used to enhance, and not replace, the healing that primarily comes from the sound of the gong.

One benefit in using these methodologies is that the client may continue to use them for days or weeks after the session to reinforce and integrate the healing that occurred during the playing of the gong.

Over time and practice, the gong therapist will become familiar with the effectiveness of the various methodologies and can more easily incorporate them seamlessly into the therapy sessions.

Asanas: The Body Positions of Gong Therapy

In the practice of yoga, the physical postures, or *asanas*, are instrumental in creating a state of consciousness and mental attitude in the practitioner. Some postures are activating, others are relaxing, and some induce an automatic state of meditation.

Similarly, the posture, or more specifically the physical position of the client during the therapy session, significantly influences the experience and effects created by the sound of the gong.

In theory, a gong therapy session could be conducted with the client in a seated position. However, most therapeutic environments (massage therapy, chiropractic, acupuncture, and some forms of psychotherapy), require that the client be lying down. Reclining postures are usually conducive to relaxation and receptivity to the therapy and can be assumed by most clients, whether the position is on a massage table, bed, couch, or floor.

For reclining postures, a massage table is ideal for gong therapy although the floor may also be used, particularly if it is desired for the client to assume a restorative yoga posture or asana to enhance the effects of the session as described later in this chapter. In some cases, a bed or couch may be used but these may inhibit the optimal positioning of the gongs.

The client may either relax on the back (supine relaxation) or on the stomach (prone relaxation). Each position brings certain benefits as well as challenges for the client as described here.

Supine Relaxation

Supine relaxation is done by lying on the back, face up, with the arms relaxed by the sides and usually with the palms turned up (although the hands may be turned down for those with shoulder issues). In yoga this position is known as *shavasana* or Corpse Pose and is by far the most common position used in gong therapy.

Supine relaxation is often preferred because it allows for easy breathing and also allows the client to have contact with the outer environment in the face-up position in order to create a sense of security and connection with the therapist. For many clients this is a familiar posture that encourages relaxation.

A drawback to this position is that the client may be inclined to open the eyes to see what the therapist is doing and this can detract from the inner experience of the therapeutic sound. Another problem with this posture is that for some people lying flat on the back is uncomfortable due to low back or hip problems. For these people, a **supported supine position** can be accomplished by placing some support (rolled blanket, cushion, yoga bolster) under the knees, or simply allowing the client to rest with knees bent and feet flat.

For women in the later stages of pregnancy, this position can be modified by relaxing on the side.

Prone Relaxation

Prone relaxation is done by lying on the stomach, face down, with the head either turned to one side or with the hands folded under head so that breathing can easily occur. If a massage table is used with an opening for the face and nose, arms can be resting by the sides of the body. A small support cushion can be placed under the forehead to allow for easy breathing.

While this position is not often used in gong therapy, it may be beneficial to create a deeper state of withdrawal from the outer environment, as well as to facilitate healing on the backside of the body, or when it is more comfortable to rest on the stomach instead of the back.

Restorative Yoga Postures

In addition to supine or prone relaxation on the floor or massage table, the client may also be placed in a supported or restorative yoga posture to allow for a deeper opening or releasing in specific areas of the body. The yoga postures are also helpful for creating an emotional attitude or a psychological state in the client and enable and direct the flow of energy or prana more precisely.

There are several asanas or physical positions a gong therapy client can assume, depending upon the desired effect of the therapy session and the ability of the client or environment to support the posture. Blankets, bolsters, cushions or other supportive props are required for these positions and it is important to take time to insure that the client is completely comfortable with the placement of the support props.

Almost any restorative or supported yoga posture may be used in the therapy session, provided that the client can remain relaxed in the posture for part or all of the gong playing portion of the therapy session. In some cases, the yoga asana or posture can be released after the initial playing of the gong and the client is allowed to assume a supine or prone relaxation position for the remainder of the session.

Three suggested and effective yoga restorative postures for a gong therapy session are (1) Supported Child Pose, (2) Supported Hip Openers, and (3) Supported Heart Opener.

Supported Child Pose (Salamba Balasana)

How to Do It: Sitting on the heels, fold forward over a stack of folded blankets or a bolster so the head and chest are supported off the floor. Turn the head so the neck is comfortable. Relax and allow the breath to move deeply into the body.

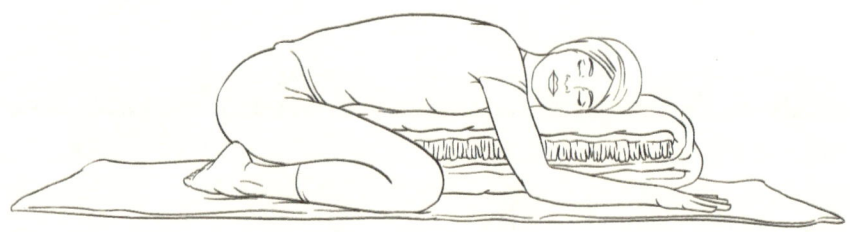

Benefits: The grounding and nurturing nature of this posture calms anxiety, reduces stress, and supports the vital energy centers of the stomach, head and heart. It allows for the release of protective holding in the abdominal area and improves digestion and elimination. It is helpful for radiating nerve pain and difficulties with the bladder and bowels.

Supported Hip Openers (Supta Baddha Konasana)

How to Do It: Sitting on the floor, bring the soles of the feet together and let the knees fall open to the sides. Place folded blankets or blocks under the knees to support the hips. Place a bolster under the back if you desire and slowly lower the back to the floor. Let the arms fall open to the sides. Relax and allow the breath to move across the hips.

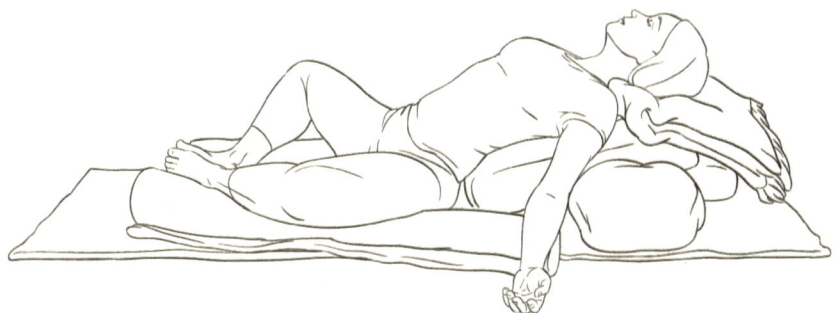

Benefits: The posture soothes the sympathetic nervous system, calms anxiety, reduces stress, improves focus, reduces tension and relieves headaches. Other benefits include easing menstrual cramps, supporting fertility and pregnancy, improving digestion, and increasing flexibility in the inner hips and groins.

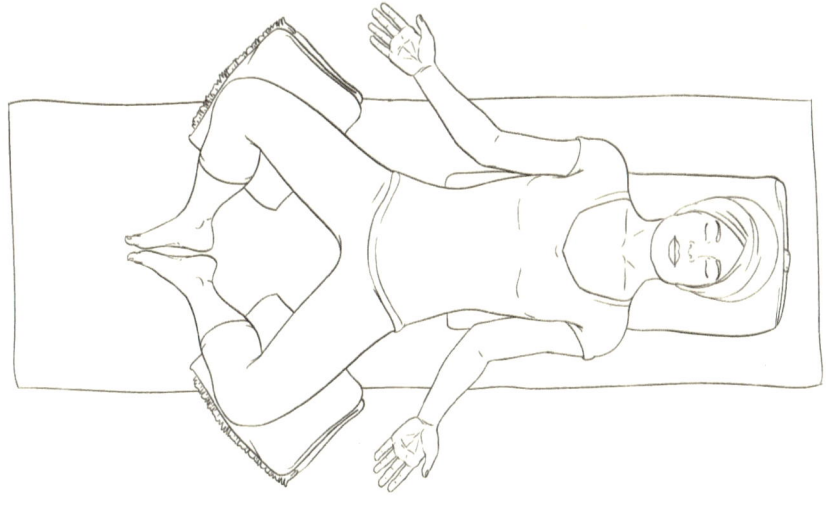

Supported Heart Opener (Supta Anahata Chakra)

How to Do It: Lying on the floor, place folded blankets or a bolster under the knees to support the hips. Place a rolled blanket below the shoulders so the heart is lifted and another rolled blanket under the neck to support the head. Let the arms fall open above your shoulders, elbows comfortably bent. Relax and allow the breath to move through the heart.

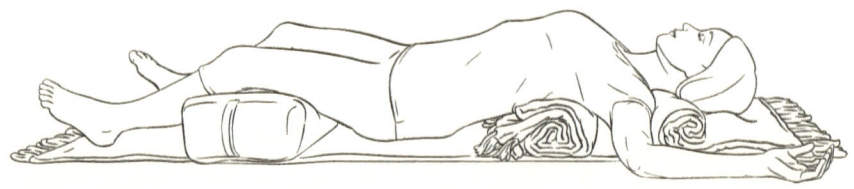

Benefits: The posture aids in releasing tension in the jaw, neck, shoulders and upper back. It increases the lung capacity, activates the thymus gland and stimulates the body's immune function. It can aid in releasing grief, sadness, and shame and opens the possibilities of creating healthy emotional relationships and balancing boundaries between the self and others.

Consider the Client

Ultimately the body position, or asana, used during the therapy session should be comfortable for the client according to their abilities and physical condition. While the position may be changed, ideally it is comfortable enough to be maintained throughout the session. Large movements, such as sitting up or moving the head, interrupt the flow of the healing energy and create a distraction from the experience.

While you may feel that a particular position is more beneficial than another, always ask the client before the gong is played if they feel comfortable enough to relax in that position during the gong playing session.

Drishtis: Role of the Eyes in Gong Therapy

The eyes direct our movements, intention and consciousness. We are drawn to what our eyes see, and our ability to manifest and transform depends upon our ability to see and hold in our sight what we desire to have and where we wish to go.

The eyes play an important role in the experience of all therapeutic endeavors. For example, some types of therapy require that the eyes be held open and focused on an object or an activity, such as physical therapy and art therapy. Other therapeutic approaches are best facilitated with eyes closed, such as music therapy and some forms of hypnotherapy. There are also therapeutic practices that allow the client to have the eyes either open or closed, such as massage therapy and psychotherapy.

In yoga therapy, the eyes are also involved in the healing process through the focusing of the eyes (either open or closed) on specific areas within or outside of the body. These gazes, or eye positions, in yoga therapy are called *drishtis* and they are also used in gong therapy.

Relaxed Eye Positions

The drishtis where the client maintains a relaxed gaze with the eyes either opened, covered, slightly open, or fully closed are the easiest for clients who may have not experienced using directed gazes in the practice of yoga or meditation.

Here are the effects and recommendations for holding the eyes in the various relaxed positions:

Eyes Open

When the eyes are open during a gong therapy session, the attention is directed outward from the inner experience and the sympathetic nervous system is dominant. This creates a state of alertness and activates the left side of the brain and the rational, analytical mind.

Open eyes are recommended for clients who are feeling "out of the body" and disoriented in time or space. Open eyes may also be beneficial for clients with trust issues and heightened anxiety around new experiences. Open eyes are always best for children, and helpful for clients who may experience dizziness while resting on the back.

Eyes Partially Open (1/10th open)

When the eyes are partially open with the eyelids relaxed (approximately 9/10th closed to allow only a small amount of light to enter), there is a calming and balancing effect on the mind. This creates openness to experiencing the effects of the session without completely shutting down the sympathetic nervous system.

Eyes partially open are recommended when there is an interaction occurring between the therapist and client, such as giving instructions or asking for feedback from the client. Eyes partially open are also helpful when the purpose of the session is to activate the meditative mind or to work with intuition.

Eyes Covered

When the eyes are covered with an eye pillow or towel, there is a deep quieting of the nervous system and sensory input is greatly reduced. This allows for a deeper inward experience and facilitates the yogic state of pratyahara, or sensory withdrawal and synchronization.

Eyes covered are recommended for regression therapy or when dealing with past traumas. Eyes covered are also helpful to slow down an overactive mind and engender a sense of security.

Eyes Fully Closed

When the eyes are fully closed during a gong therapy session, the attention is directed inward and the parasympathetic nervous system becomes dominant. This creates a state of relaxation and activates the right side of the brain and the sensing or intuitive mind.

Fully closed eyes are recommended for clients who are comfortable with their surroundings and ready to relax deeply. Fully closed eyes are also recommended when using directed eye gazes on the drishti points to create additional therapeutic effects as explained in the next section.

Directed Eye Positions: The Drishti Points

In yoga, a drishti, or eye position, aids in directing prana and transferring energy to where the gaze of the eyes is directed. The specific focus area of the gaze is called a *drishti point*, and these drishti points are uniquely effective in transferring prana to heal the body, balance the mind, and transform consciousness.

During a gong therapy session, when the client focuses on a certain area in the body, or drishti point, the sound of the gong localizes around this point to create a specific beneficial effect.

For clients who find focusing on specific drishti points difficult or uncomfortable, they may simply keep the eyes open, covered, or slightly closed without a specific focus.

Drishti Points and Effects

Holding the gaze on the various drishti points affect the parasympathetic nervous system by activating the third cranial nerve, or the optic nerve, and create a deeper sense of relaxation during a gong therapy session. The gaze should feel relaxed and not tightly held.

Crown of the Head

When the focus is directed to the crown, or slightly above the top of the head, the pineal gland is activated and there is a sensation of elevation. The higher energy centers of the brain are opened and there is an experience of transcending the physical realm.

Focusing on the crown of the head during a gong therapy session is helpful for dealing with depression and sadness. It increases the connection to the spiritual realm and can be helpful when transitioning through major life changes. Pain relief can also be obtained as the boundaries of the physical body are transcended.

Brow Point

When the focus is directed to the brow point (third eye), or slightly above the two eyebrows, the pituitary gland is activated and intuition is heightened. There is a sense of peace and stillness.

Focusing at the brow point can be helpful in dealing with glandular disorders and also to access inner guidance or intuition. The focus is useful in balancing the polarities of the body and mind and can aid in resolving gender confusion, as well as developing a relationship to the hidden side of the self.

Tip of Nose

When the focus is directed toward the tip of the nose, the frontal lobe of brain is strengthened and concentration is enhanced. This focus creates new energy pathways in the body and modifies patterns in the brain.

Focusing at the tip of the nose during the gong therapy session helps with attention deficit disorder. It can also be useful for improving memory and concentration, as well as dealing with obsessive-compulsive disorders.

Bottom of Chin

When the focus is directed toward the bottom of the chin, the emotional body is affected. The result is a cooling, calming, and centering of the emotions.

This focus is good for dealing with emotional disorders and upsets, and to reduce hypersensitivity and paranoia.

Soft Palate of Mouth

When the focus is directed to the soft palate, or back roof of the mouth, the rhythms of the autonomic nervous system are balanced and the parasympathetic and sympathetic nervous systems are integrated. This results in a lowering of stress, strengthening the immune system function, and creating a sense of happiness and emotional wellbeing. The distribution of the blood flow is also improved, as well as blood circulation, hormonal release, heart rate, thermoregulation, urination, bowel activity, and appetite.

To aid in this focus, the top of the tongue can be allowed to float and relax at the back of the roof of the mouth

The focus on the soft palate of the mouth during a therapy session is helpful for re-establishing the normal daily biorhythm cycles and consequently good for such conditions as jet lag and bipolar disorder. The focus on this area of the body is recommended when dealing with depression or mood episodes, and is especially effective when working with the emotional body. Due to its beneficial effect on the immune system, it is also effective when dealing with allergies, viruses, and susceptibility to illness. On a subtle level, this focus also strengthens the auric field.

Palms of the Hands

Focusing on the open palms of the hands during a gong therapy session increases receptivity and openness to change. It also aids in facilitating the reception of intuitive information and increases the healing energy of the hands.

This focus is recommended to still the thinking mind and increase sensitivity to feeling the energy field around the body. It is helpful in dealing with issues of self-trust, paranoia, and interpersonal connectivity.

Soles of the Feet

Focusing on the soles of the feet during a gong therapy session develops the sensation of embodiment and experience of the protective magnetic field of the earth.

This focus is helpful to bring people back into their body and to reduce spaciness and alienation.

Base of the Spine

Focusing on the base of the spine during a gong therapy session can aid in the awakening of the kundalini energy.

This focus is suggested for people who may be experiencing energy blocks or a disconnection from their instinctual self.

Pelvic Area

Focusing on the pelvic area during a gong therapy session can balance emotional and sexual energy.

This focus can be used by people who may be over emotional or do not have the capacity for emotional intimacy. In some cases, it may be useful for those who have experienced sexual abuse or difficulties connected to childbirth.

Navel Point Area

Focusing on the navel point during a gong therapy session creates a strong sense of self and presence in the moment.

This focus is useful for people who feel disempowered, overwhelmed, or fearful.

Heart Area

Focusing on the heart area during a gong therapy session creates self-compassion, acceptance, and balance.

This focus is helpful for healing the emotional body and expanding the sense of self.

Throat Area

Focusing on the throat area during a gong therapy session enhances the ability to hear what needs to be heard and to say what needs to be said.

This focus allows for recognition of our limiting internal dialogues and the patterns of communication that do not serve us.

The Most Important Drishti

The most important gaze is one that allows the client to relax and go deeper into the experience of the healing session. Always give permission to relax the gaze during the session, and to discontinue if there is any discomfort or disorientation. Create an atmosphere of trust and permission so that whatever gaze is used, the client feels empowered to release or change it as desired.

Mudras: Hand Positions in Gong Therapy

Mudras are finger and hand positions, such as touching the tip of the thumb to the tip of the index finger, that are held during an exercise or meditation.

The hand and finger positions of mudras make important connections in the nervous system and stimulate specific energy pathways. It is said that mudras increase energy and blood circulation to different parts of the brain and to important nerve junctures and the glands. They affect the sympathetic and parasympathetic nervous systems as well as the involuntary physiological processes of the body. They are part of the Ayurvedic healing system used in India, as well as an essential part of yoga practice to regulate the breath, focus the mind and transform consciousness.

In essence, mudras are psychophysiological hand positions that rebalance the underlying energy structure of the body that is responsible for the maintenance of health and the quality of our thoughts.

By curling, stretching, crossing and touching fingers to other fingers and areas of the hand we can effectively talk to the body and mind. Each finger has a quality that it represents and stimulates. The fingers are connected to the elements of the body, the chakras, the major organs, and even planetary energies. The hand is an energy map of consciousness as well as a mapping of the entire body and its functions.

There are hundreds of mudras and their use has been documented in India for centuries and more recently in the Western world. They are an essential part of Gong Therapy and we have selected some of the most effective ones to be used. Any mudra, however, can be incorporated into a Gong Therapy session and its use with the sound of the gong accelerates its healing properties.

To begin using mudras in a gong therapy session, select the simple ones and familiarize yourself with the properties of the major mudras presented in this section. There are tables of mudras and their properties at the end of this section to help you select ones that will be helpful for your client.

Mudras are essentially benign in nature, with few contraindications, and may be used by people of all ages and all backgrounds. The primary consideration is that the mudra be comfortable for the person to hold and that you give permission to the client to release it during the session if so desired.

If the mudra feels supportive and helpful to the client, then encourage them to continue practicing it after the session, holding it for as much as 30 to 45 minutes a day, divided into smaller periods of practice if they wish.

Gyan Mudra (Jnana Mudra)

Benefits - Energizes the brain, promotes creativity, develops intelligence, empowers the nervous system, reduces mental tension, creates a positive effect on the emotions.

Technique - Touch the tip of the index finger to the tip of the thumb. For Gong Yoga therapy, use both hands and relax them beside the body.

Traditional Ayurvedic Treatment - Alzheimer's disease, acne, cerebral palsy, drowsiness, high blood pressure, dementia, retinal degeneration, diabetes, depression, all endocrine gland disorders, weak heart, heat intolerance, multiple sclerosis, excessive mucus, nervous system disorders, excessive sleep as well as sleeplessness, and general weakness.

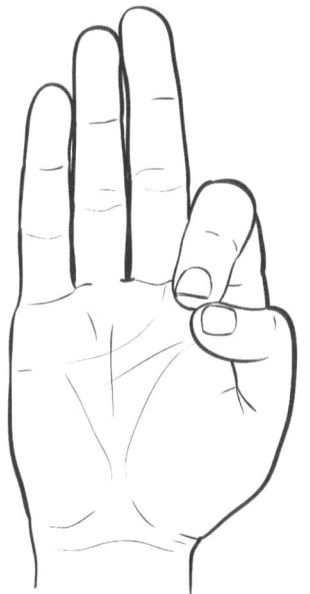

- Brings ultimate knowledge of all things
- Activates the air element and the mental realm
- Increases Jupiter energy
- Balances knowledge body (Vijnanomaya kosha)

Akasha Mudra (Shani Mudra)

Benefits - Aids in meditation, replaces negative emotions with positive thoughts, develops patience, enhances intuition, eliminates metabolic wastes and detoxifies the body.

Technique - Touch the thumb tip to the middle finger. Extend the other fingers. For Gong Yoga therapy, use both hands and relax them beside the body.

Traditional Ayurvedic Treatment - Feeling of heaviness or fullness in the body, congestion, toxicity, migraine headaches, sinusitis, strengthens bones and heart, high blood pressure, and irregular heartbeat.

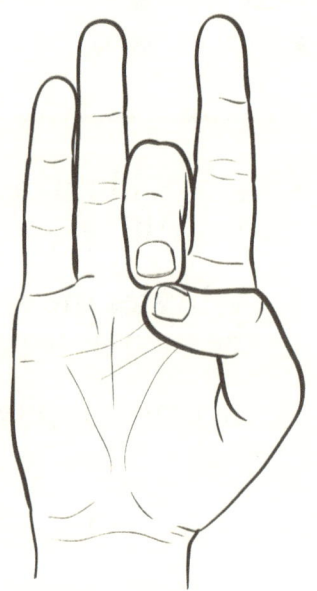

- Increases the ether (space or akash) element
- Expands consciousness
- Activates Saturn energy
- Balances the Manomaya Kosha
- Aids the Vishuddhi (Fifth) Chakra

Prithvi Mudra (Earth Mudra)

Benefits - Increases vitality, strength, and endurance. Builds and invigorates bones, cartilage, skin, hair, nails, tendons and internal organs. Strengthens digestion and assimilation. Promotes adaptability to change and restores trust and equilibrium.

Technique - Touch the thumb tip to the tip of the ring finger. Extend the other fingers. For Gong Yoga therapy, use both hands and relax them beside the body.

Traditional Ayurvedic Treatment - Chronic fatigue, tiredness, emaciation, fractures, atrophied muscles, dry skin, ulcers, fever, jaundice, loss of smell, vitamin deficiency.

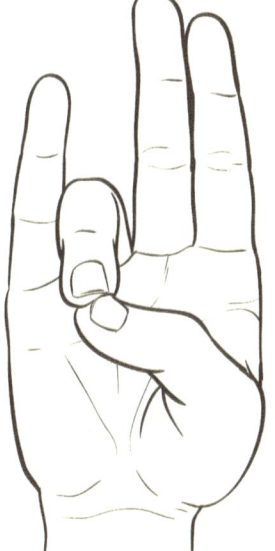

- Balances & normalizes the earth element
- Stabilizes the first chakra
- Builds tolerance & patience
- Creates centeredness & grounding

Varuna Mudra (Budhi or Mercury Mudra)

Benefits - Decreases dryness, enhances physical beauty, maintains equilibrium in the fluid balance of the body. Improves communication, balances emotions.

Technique - Touch the thumb tip to the tip of the little finger. Extend the other fingers. For Gong Yoga therapy, use both hands and relax them beside the body.

Traditional Ayurvedic Treatment - Loss of taste, dryness of eyes, dehydration, indigestion constipation, dryness of skin, hormone deficiency, and degeneration of joint-cartilage.

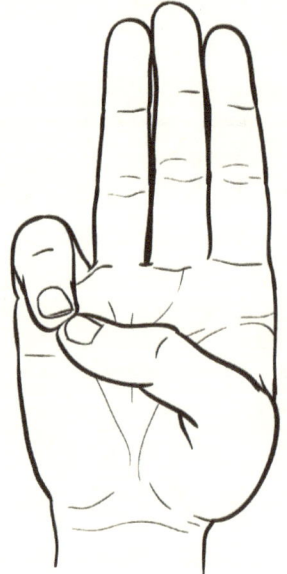

- Increases and balances the water (jal) element
- Improves communication
- Maintains equilibrium
- Improves joint health

Vayu Mudra (Wind Mudra)

Benefits - Calms restlessness and soothes the mind. Sedates an overactive nervous system. Relaxes tense muscles.

Technique - Touch the index finger to the base of the thumb and hold the index finger down. Extend the other fingers. For Gong Yoga therapy, use both hands and relax them beside the body.

Traditional Ayurvedic Treatment - Muscular trembling, sciatica, excessive gas, gout, palsy, rheumatism, sleeplessness, stress, anxiety, indecisiveness, hormonal imbalances, tinnitus, dizziness, breathlessness, muscle spasms, constipation and joint pain.

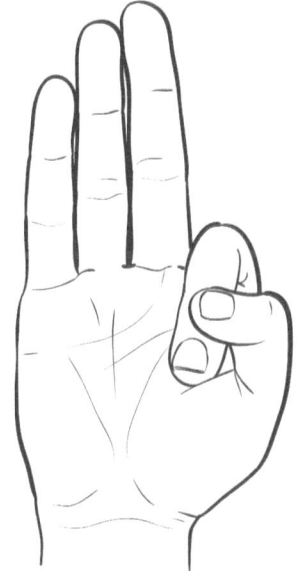

- Decreases the air element
- Soothes the mind
- Calms restlessness
- Reduces Vata dosha

Shunya Mudra (Sky Mudra)

Benefits - Improves hearing and increases appreciation of sound. Aids in maintaining balance. Reduces the sense of being "spaced out" or disconnected from reality.

Technique - Touch the middle finger to the base of the thumb and lock the finger down with the thumb. Extend the other fingers. For Gong Yoga therapy, use both hands and relax them beside the body.

Traditional Ayurvedic Treatment - Deafness, tinnitus, earache, vertigo, emptiness or numbness in the body, low blood pressure.

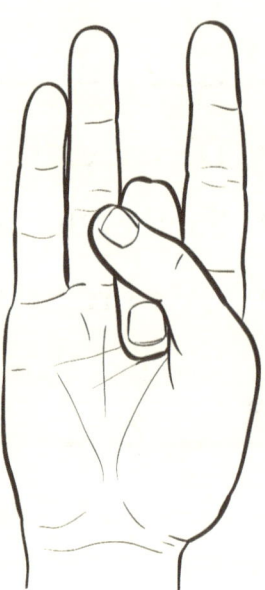

- Decreases the ether (space or akash) element
- Reduces vata (spaciness)
- Improves hearing
- Maintains balance

Surya Mudra (Sun Mudra)

Benefits - Maintains body temperature and proper metabolism. Strengthens digestion, reduces fat, detoxifies the body. Reduces fatigue, depression, and mental heaviness.

Technique - Touch the ring finger to the base of the thumb and lock the finger down with the thumb. Extend the other fingers. For Gong Yoga therapy, use both hands and relax them beside the body.

Traditional Ayurvedic Treatment - Low body temperature, intolerance to cold, underactive thyroid gland, obesity, loss of appetite, cataracts, poor vision, weak digestion, loss of appetite, blocked breathing, constipation, and high cholesterol.

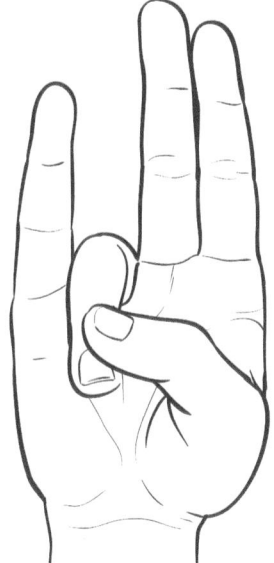

- Increases the fire element
- Decreases the earth element
- Maintains body temperature
- Detoxifies the body

Jalodamshaka Mudra (Water Reducing Mudra)

Benefits - Aids in all conditions created by a water imbalance in the body. Especially effective for people with a kapha-pitta constitution. Can relieve mental pain, a sense of emotional heaviness, depression and excessive emotionality.

Technique - Touch the little finger at the base of the thumb and hold the finger down gently with the thumb. For Gong Yoga therapy, use both hands and relax them beside the body.

Traditional Ayurvedic Treatment – Edema (water retention), watery eyes, excessive salivation, running nose, excess of hormones, cold and clammy hands and feet, hyperacidity, excessive urination, throat pain and obesity.

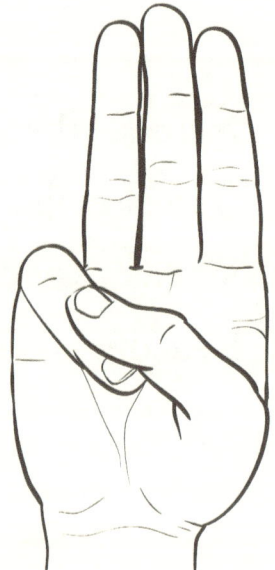

- Reduces the water element
- Good for kapha-pitta constitution
- Relieves mental pain
- Reduces emotional heaviness

Prana Mudra (Vitality Mudra)

Benefits - Improves circulation, moderates blood pressure, strengthens the heart, increases vitality, aids in recovery and immunity, reduces fatigue, improves eyesight, strengthens willpower and confidence, sedates the mind and relaxes the body.

Technique - Touch the thumb tip to the tips of the ring finger and little finger. Extend the index and middle finger. For Gong Yoga therapy, use both hands and relax them beside the body.

Traditional Ayurvedic Treatment - Chronic fatigue, weakened immunity, intolerance to heat and stress, hyperthyroidism, sleeplessness, high blood pressure, rheumatoid arthritis, allergies, colitis, menopause symptoms, skin rashes, jaundice, sore throat, premature aging.

- Stabilizes & calms
- Increases energy reserves
- Complements all other mudras
- Activates the first chakra and pelvic floor.

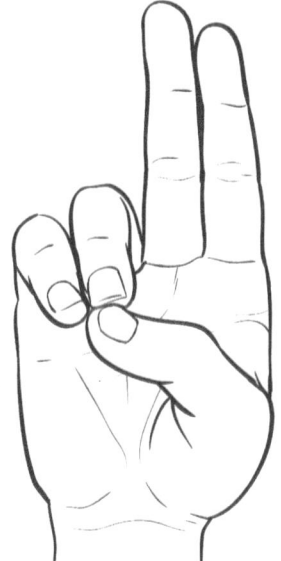

Apana Mudra (Elimination Mudra)

Benefits - Purifies and energizes the body. Improves elimination on all levels. Enhances balance, harmony, patience, and the ability to envision. Gives courage for new beginnings. Promotes mental clarity, the clearing of negative emotions, and the development of *saucha* (purity of thought and action).

Technique - Touch the thumb to the tips of the middle finger and ring finger. Extend the index and little finger. For Gong Yoga therapy, use both hands and relax them beside the body.

Traditional Ayurvedic Treatment - Constipation, burning sensation, hemorrhoids, obstruction of urine, bladder and uterus problems, liver and gall bladder dysfunction, skin rashes, cervical spondylosis, diabetes, dry skin and hair, detoxification, debility, dysentery, flu, joint pains, kidney problems, nausea, osteoarthritis, weakness, and delayed childbirth. (Usually recommended during the last month of pregnancy but not the prior months.)

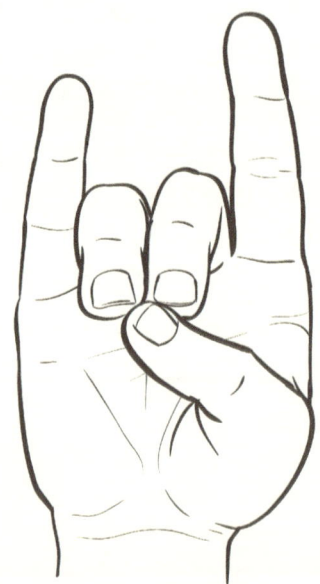

- Regulates downward moving energy of the body
- Decreases pitta
- Purifies and energizes
- Develops *saucha*

Apana Vayu Mudra
(Mritsamjivani "Life Saving" Mudra)

Benefits - Improves circulation, moderates blood pressure, strengthens the heart, increases vitality, sedates the mind and relaxes the body.

Technique - Place the tip of the index finger to the base of the thumb. Touch the thumb tip to the middle and ring finger. For Gong Yoga therapy, use both hands and relax them beside the body.

Traditional Ayurvedic Treatment - Heart attack, chest pains, heart palpitations, high blood pressure, arthritis, appendicitis, abdominal pain, kidney ailments, nausea, intense acute pain such as headaches, toothaches, backaches, and all joint pains.

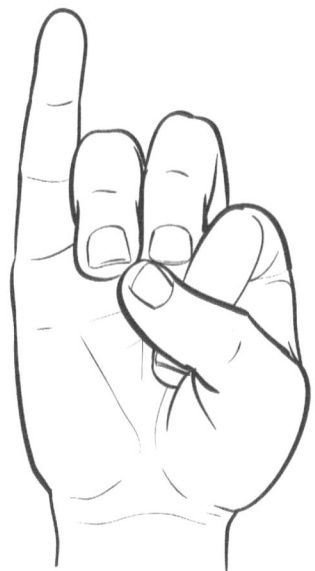

- Promotes self-nurturing
- Creates healthy boundaries in relationships
- Improves circulation
- Strengthens heart

Vata Nashak Mudra
(Air and Space Reducing Mudra)

Benefits - Aids in grounding, reduces spaciness, and scattered thinking. Benefits those with a vata constitution.

Technique – Place the tips of the index and middle finger at the base of the thumb and press them gentle down with the thumb. For Gong Yoga therapy, use both hands and relax them beside the body.

Traditional Ayurvedic Treatment – Lack of stamina, chronic fatigue, poor memory, indecisiveness, sleeplessness, emaciation, cold intolerance, numbness, dry skin, hair and nails, painful joints, and most painful conditions (headache, earache, throat pain, heel pain, joint pain, toothache, etc.).

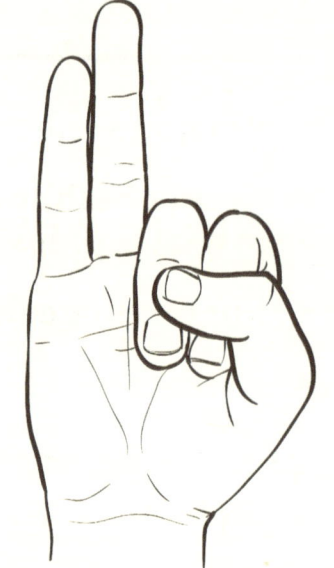

- Decreases the elements of air and ether in the body
- Decreases vata
- Aids in grounding
- Improves memory

Linga Mudra (Fire Mudra)

Benefits – Increases will power, self-confidence and focus. Strengthens sense of self and identity. Increases heat in the body and overcomes lethargy and laziness.

Technique – Interlace the four fingers with the right little finger on the bottom. Extend the right thumb sticking up and circle the left thumb around the base of the right thumb and touch the tip of the left index finger. For Gong Yoga therapy, hold the mudra relaxed on the abdomen.

Traditional Ayurvedic Treatment – Relieves shivering, chills, cold and flu symptoms. Increases beneficial fever to burn away impurities. Used for weight loss, sore throat and respiratory ailments caused by change of weather. Helpful for asthma and over production of mucus or phlegm. Overcoming sexual debility in males.

- Increases fire element and pitta humor
- Improves thyroid, parathyroid, liver and pancreas
- Increases focus

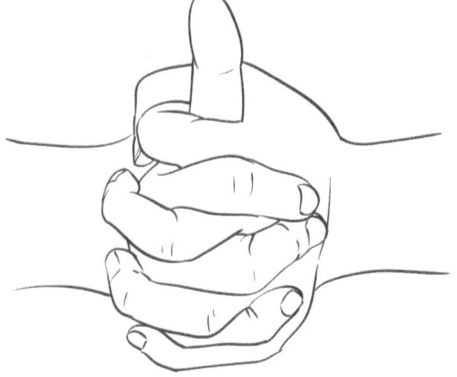

Shakti Mudra (Goddess Mudra)

Benefits – Calms the mind, brings about sleep, reduces cramping and pelvic tension, heals emotional and physical trauma around sexual abuse, increases sense of intimacy and femininity. Promotes peaceful feelings and connection with divine goddess energy.

Technique - Touch the tips of the ring and little finger of both hands together and extend them upward. Fold the index and middle fingers around the thumbs and press the thumb gently into the palm. For Gong Yoga therapy, relax the hands on the chest near the bottom of the rib cage.

Traditional Ayurvedic Treatment – Reduce spasms of pelvic and intestine area, menstrual complaints, sleeplessness, emotional upset, and uneven breath rate.

- Connects with divine goddess
- Relaxes the intestines and pelvic muscles.
- Calms Mind
- Regulates respiratory activity above the stomach, in the lower chest area.

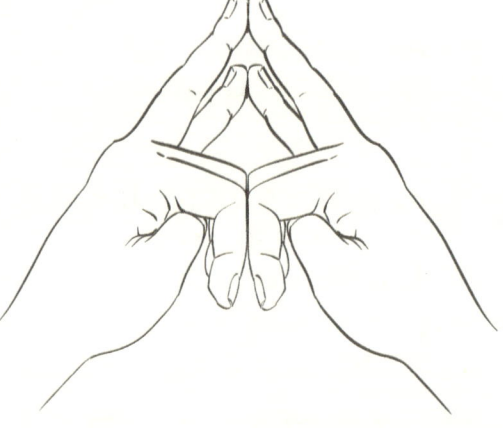

Matanga Mudra (Elephant Mudra)

Benefits – Brings peace of mind, strengthens digestion, reduces mental tension, enhances diaphragmatic breathing, improves the ability to communicate, and fosters a sense of innocence and self-trust.

Technique – Interlace the fingers with the right little finger on the bottom and the left thumb over the right thumb. Extend the middle fingers and press them together from base to tip. Hold the mudra in a relaxed fashion over the solar plexus with the fingers pointing out.

Traditional Ayurvedic Treatment – Indigestion, gall bladder and liver dysfunction, kidney problems, irregular breathing, diabetes, jaw tension and pain or Temporomandibular Joint Syndrome (*TMJ*).

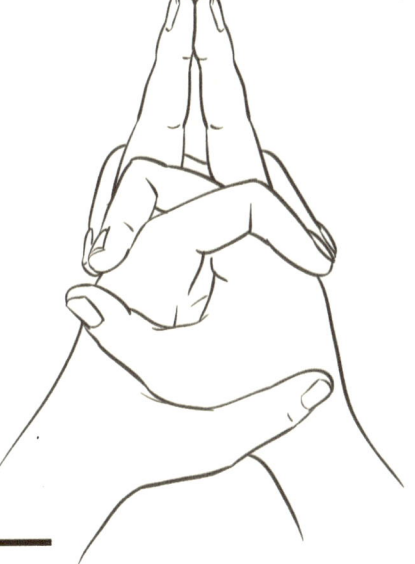

- Activates the earth and space elements
- Balances the heart, liver, kidneys and gall bladder
- Gives enormous strength like an elephant.
- Brings peace of mind

Bhramara Mudra (Bee Mudra)

Benefits - Balances and strengthens the immune system. Reduces environmental sensitivity and allergic reactions. Improves health of the lungs. Aids thymus gland functioning. Strengthens the heart chakra and supports healthy boundaries in relationships.

Technique - Touch the tip of the index finger to the base of the thumb. Touch the thumb to the middle finger between the side of the fingernail and the first joint. Extend the ring and little finger. For Gong Yoga therapy, use both hands and relax them beside the body, or over the lap palms up.

Traditional Ayurvedic Treatment – Allergies, coughing, congestion, asthma, sinusitis, and burning sensation in lungs.

- Creates harmony between the inner and outer environment
- Strengthens immune system
- Reduces allergic reactions
- Strengthens heart chakra

Kshepana Mudra (Ambrosia Mudra)

Benefits – Relieves inner tension and eliminates negative energies of the body. Strengthens the function of the large intestine, lungs and skin.

Technique – Interlace the fingers of both hands and cross the left thumb over the right finger. Extend the index fingers and flatten against each other. For Gong Yoga Therapy, relax the hands on the body with the index fingers pointing toward the feet.

Traditional Ayurvedic Treatment – Constipation, skin disorders, lung congestion (improves exhalation), emphysema, paranoia, and chronic tension.

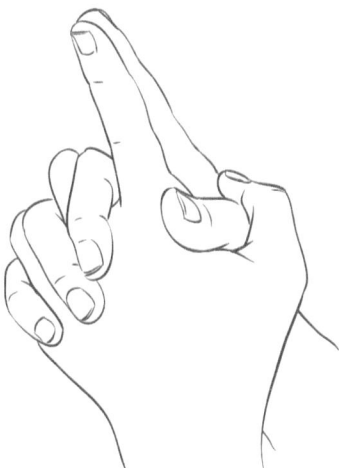

- Increases the flow of energy in and out of the body
- Empties out needless thoughts and expended feelings
- Relieves inner tension
- Strengthens large intestine, lungs, and skin

Kubera Mudra (Prosperity Mudra)

Benefits –Overcomes tiredness, brings peace of mind, promotes alertness and confidence so that opportunities to be recognized and acted upon.

Technique - Touch the tips of the thumb, index finger, and middle finger together. Curl the ring finger and little finger into the palm or allow them to relax free. For Gong Yoga therapy, relax both hands by the body

Traditional Ayurvedic Treatment – Sleeplessness, fatigue, loss of the sense of smell. Balances the flow of breath equally through both nostrils and clears the sinuses.

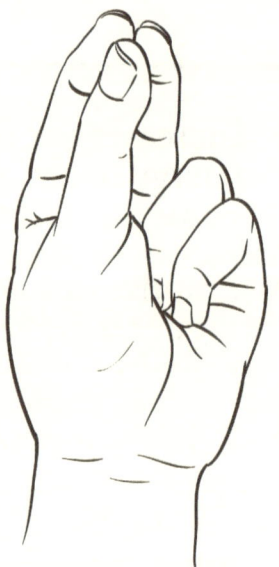

- Opens the flow of prosperity and abundance
- Overcomes tiredness
- Brings peace of mind
- Promotes alertness and confidence

Yoni Mudra (Tantric Mudra)

Benefits – Balances the sexual and spiritual energies of the practitioner. Invites sacredness into rituals and practices and connects to the divine feminine principle. Strengthens inhalation and functioning of the nervous system.

Technique - Open the index fingers and thumbs of both hands wide apart and touch the tips of thumb and tips of the index fingers together, creating a triangle. Curl the remaining fingers into the hands. For Gong Yoga therapy, this mudra may be: 1) Held relaxed against the heart with the index finger pointing up which is the masculine expression of this mudra, or 2) Held relaxed over the pelvis with the index fingers pointing down which is the feminine expression.

Traditional Ayurvedic Treatment – Irregularity and pain of the menstrual cycles, post-menopausal difficulties, stomach pain, easing childbirth.

- Harmonizes the flow of energy between the second and fourth chakras
- Invites sacredness
- Connects to divine feminine
- Strengthens inhalation

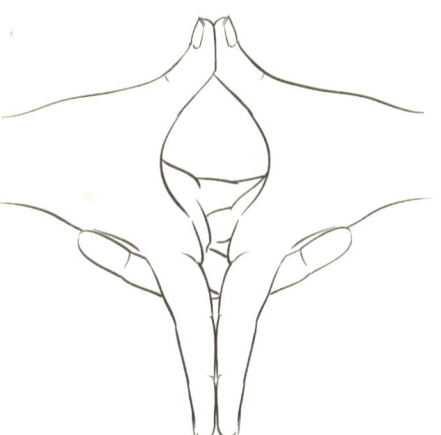

Rudra Mudra (Solar Plexus Mudra)

Benefits - Strengthens stomach, spleen and pancreas. Improves digestion and assimilation. Helps organ prolapses. Creates inner resolve, strength, and sense of personal power and manifestation.

Technique - Touch the thumb tip to the index finger and ring finger. Extend the other fingers. For Gong Yoga therapy, use both hands and relax them on top of thighs, palms up.

Traditional Ayurvedic Treatment - Emaciation, dizziness, fatigue, low vitality, impaired digestion, and weakness.

- Centering and empowering
- Increases earth element
- Balances third chakra
- Improves digestion

Kaleshvara Mudra (Lord of Time Mudra)

Benefits – Improves concentration and memory function. Aids in eliminating bad habits, addictive behavior, and negative feelings. Calms the mind, strengthens the heart, and supports self-reflection.

Technique – Touch the tips of the middle fingers together and extend them outward. Bend the other three fingers toward the palms and join them together at the middle joint. Touch the tips of the thumbs together. For Gong Yoga therapy, relax the thumbs against the heart.

Traditional Ayurvedic Treatment – Memory loss, attention deficit disorder (scattered thinking), addictions, weakness of heart and pericardium.

- Activates the elements of fire and ether

- Calms mind

- Eliminates addictive behavior

- Improves concentration

Hakini Mudra (Third Eye Mudra)

Benefits – Improves memory, increases perception, integrates the hemispheres of the brain, balances the five elements, and deepens respiration.

Technique - Touch the tips of the fingers and thumbs together. Allow the little fingers and thumbs to pull slightly away from the other three fingers. For Gong Yoga therapy, allow the hands to relax on the body.

Traditional Ayurvedic Treatment – Memory loss, irregular breathing, bipolar episodes.

- Actives the sixth chakra and frontal lobe of the brain
- Improves memory
- Balances the five elements
- Increases perception

Ushas Mudra (Venus Lock Mudra)

Benefits – Facilitates mental alertness and creativity, supports new beginnings in life. Increases the pleasure response and zest for life.

Technique – Interlace the two hands so that the right thumb is on to for men and the left thumb on top for women. The inside thumb presses on the web of the opposite thumb. The outside thumb presses on the outside mound of the other thumb.

Traditional Ayurvedic Treatment – Sexual dysfunction, hormonal imbalance, gender identity confusion, dull mind upon awakening.

- Channels and refines sexual and creative energy
- Facilitates mental alertness
- Supports new beginnings
- Increases pleasure response

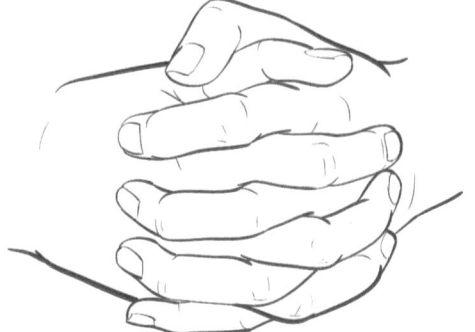

Mudras for Symptoms and Disease

MUDRA	TRADITIONAL TREATMENT
GYAN	Alzheimer's disease, acne, cerebral palsy, high blood pressure, dementia, retinal degeneration, diabetes, depression, endocrine gland disorders, heat intolerance, multiple sclerosis, excessive mucus, ANS disorders, drowsiness, weak heart, excessive sleep, sleeplessness, weakness
AKASHA	Feeling of heaviness or fullness in the body, congestion, toxicity, migraine headaches, sinusitis, strengthens bones and heart, high blood pressure, and irregular heartbeat
PRITHVI	Chronic fatigue, tiredness, emaciation, fractures, atrophied muscles, dry skin, ulcers, fever, jaundice, loss of smell, vitamin deficiency
VARUNA	Loss of taste, dry eyes, dehydration, indigestion constipation, dryness of skin, hormone deficiency, degeneration of joint-cartilage
VAYU	Muscular trembling, sciatica, gout, rheumatism, sleeplessness, stress, anxiety, indecisiveness, hormonal imbalances, tinnitus, dizziness, breathlessness, constipation, joint pain
SHUNYA	Deafness, tinnitus, earache, vertigo, emptiness or numbness in the body, low blood pressure
SURYA	Low body temperature, intolerance to cold, underactive thyroid, obesity, loss of appetite, cataracts, poor vision, weak digestion, blocked breathing, constipation, high cholesterol
JALODAMSHAKA	Edema (water retention), watery eyes, excessive salivation, running nose, excess of hormones, cold and clammy hands and feet, hyperacidity, excessive urination, throat pain and obesity
PRANA	Chronic fatigue, weakened immunity, heat intolerance, hyperthyroidism, sleeplessness, high blood pressure, rheumatoid arthritis, allergies, colitis, menopause symptoms, skin rashes, jaundice, sore throat, premature aging

APANA	Constipation, burning sensation, hemorrhoids, obstruction urine, bladder and uterus problems, liver and gall bladder dysfunction, skin rashes, diabetes, dry skin and hair, debility, dysentery, flu, joint pains, kidney problems, nausea, osteoarthritis, weakness, delayed childbirth
APANA VAYU	Heart attack, chest pains, heart palpitations, high blood pressure, arthritis, appendicitis, abdominal pain, kidney ailments, nausea, acute pain, toothaches, backaches, joint pains
VATA NASHAK	Lack of stamina, chronic fatigue, poor memory, indecisiveness, sleeplessness, emaciation, cold intolerance, numbness, dry skin, hair and nails, painful joints, and most painful conditions
LINGA	Chills, cold and flu symptoms. Increases beneficial fever to burn impurities. Sore throat and respiratory ailments., asthma, excessive mucus or phlegm. Male sexual debility
SHAKTI	Spasms of pelvic and intestine area, menstrual complaints, sleeplessness, emotional upset
MATANGA	Indigestion, gall bladder and liver dysfunction, kidney problems, irregular breathing, diabetes, and jaw tension and pain (*TMJ*)
BHRAMARA	Allergies, coughing, congestion, asthma, sinusitis, and burning sensation in lungs
KSHEPANA	Constipation, skin disorders, lung congestion, emphysema, paranoia, and chronic tension.
KUBERA	Sleeplessness, fatigue, loss of smell.
YONI	Irregular or painful menstruation, stomach pain, post-menopausal difficulties, easing childbirth
RUDRA	Emaciation, dizziness, fatigue, low vitality, impaired digestion, and weakness
KALESHWARA	Memory loss, attention deficit disorder, addictions, weakness of heart and pericardium
HAKINI	Memory loss, irregular breathing, bipolar
USHAS	Sexual dysfunction, hormonal imbalance, gender identity confusion, dull mind upon awakening

Mudras for Chakras, Elements and Doshas

MUDRA	CHAKRA	ELEMENT	DOSHA
GYAN	6	Air (increase)	
AKASHA	5	Ether (increase)	
PRITHVI	1	Earth (increase)	
VARUNA	5	Water (increase)	
VAYU		Air (decrease)	Vata
SHUNYA	5	Ether (decrease)	Vata
SURYA	3	Fire (increase) Earth (decrease)	Kapha
JALODAMSHAKA	2	Water (reduce)	Kapha
PRANA	1	Water (increase) Earth (increase)	Vata
APANA	1	Ether (increase) Earth (increase)	Pitta
APANA VAYU	4	Air (decrease)	
VATA NASHAK	1	Ether (decrease) Air (decrease	Vata
LINGA	3	Fire (increase)	Kapha
SHAKTI	2	Water (increase) Earth (increase)	Vata
MATANGA	2, 3	Ether (increase) Earth (increase)	Pitta
BHRAMARA	4	Air (decrease)	Vata
KSHEPANA	1, 4		
KUBERA	1, 3		
YONI	2, 4		
RUDRA	3	Earth (increase)	
KALESHWARA	4, 6	Fire (increase) Ether (increase)	Kapha
HAKINI	6		
USHAS	2		

Pranayama: Role of the Breath in Gong Therapy

In the practice of gong therapy, the gong is primarily used to energize and facilitate the movement of prana to heal the body, clear the mind and elevate the consciousness. When the client can participate in this movement and direction of prana through the practices of pranayama, or conscious breathing, the effects and benefits of the therapy session can be refined and increased.

Conscious Breathing

In the practice of yoga, and in some therapeutic modalities, breath awareness is used to bring a heightened awareness to the body and mind. Conscious breathing allows for the release of old patterns and facilitates an integration of the changes that the treatments produce.

Directing the client to create an awareness of their breath can help dissipate discomfort that may arise during the gong therapy session and also bring a focus and facilitation to the healing process.

Depending upon the client's background with breath work and yoga, the gong therapist can suggest a simple approach to using the breath during the session or offer more profound breathing techniques to amplify the gong's benefits.

All breath practices may be done for a few minutes or extended throughout the gong playing session, depending upon the ability and experience of the client and their level of comfort.

Simple Pranayama

When the session begins, have the client connect to their breath and breathe fully and consciously. Have them feel the rise and fall of the diaphragm as they breathe fully and relax into the breath. After several breaths, allow them to release control of the breath but remind them they can consciously re-connect to the breath at any time to enhance the benefits of the session, or to breathe through any blocks that may arise. Tell them to simply watch the flow of their breath, without any attempt to control it or change it. You can also breathe with them initially to connect your energy to their energy.

Directed Pranayama

The client can also actively direct the breath into any areas of the body that may need healing. With the inhale, the client breathes healing energy into the affected area and allows tension and discomfort to be released with the exhale. The effectiveness of directing the breath may be enhanced by visualizing healing light being carried on the breath.

Also see the extended visualization instructions in the Meditation section ("Point-to-Point Deep Relaxation") for guiding the breath to specific points in the body to balance the body's energies and chakras.

Ratio Breathing

If the client is comfortable in bringing the breath under conscious control, they can experiment with the following breath ratios by silently counting during the inhale and the exhale. All ratio breaths bring calmness, steadiness and focus.

Equal Balanced Breath – Inhale and exhale are equal. Clients inhale while silently counting from 1 to 5 and then exhale while counting down from 5 to 1. The equal balanced breath balances the energy and emotions and centers the practitioner in the heart.

Activating Breath – Inhale is longer than exhale. Clients inhale while silently counting from 1 to 8 and then exhale while counting down from 4 to 1. The activating breath raises energy, elevates the mood and brings vitality to the body.

Relaxing Breath – Exhale is longer than inhale. Clients inhale while silently counting from 1 to 4 and then exhale while counting down from 8 to 1. The relaxing breath releases tension, soothes the emotions and calms the mind.

Releasing Breath

The releasing breath is challenging in its complexity, but yields excellent results in opening up pranic blocks and effecting deep emotional and physical releases.

The releasing breath is a four-part cycle:

- Inhale through the nose
- Exhale through the mouth with pursed lips
- Inhale through the mouth with pursed lips
- Exhale through the nose

Continue as desired. It is important that the inhaling and exhaling through the mouth be done through slightly closed or pursed lips and not through the open mouth.

Breath Retention and Suspension

The breath may be retained or held in after inhaling and suspending or held out after exhaling. This should be done at the comfort level of the client without any sense of pressure or physical discomfort.

- Retaining the breath in builds focus and concentration and vitalizes the mind.
- Suspending the breath out releases hidden fears and deep anxieties.
- Retaining the breath in and then suspending the breath out creates calmness, patience and centeredness.

Respecting the Breath

For some clients, having them work too explicitly with the breath can create anxiety or tension unless they have a practice or experience of conscious breathing or breath control.

It is usually a good idea to wait until after the first session or even several sessions before having the client experiment with the various pranayamas. Do not mix the pranayamas in the same session.

Mantras: Affirmations and Sacred Sounds in Gong Therapy

Mantras, affirmations and other sounds can be introduced into the therapy session. If the client has prior experience with mantras, traditional Kundalini Yoga mantras or simple single-sound Ayurvedic mantras may be chanted before or repeated silently during the therapy session. Alternatively, affirmations may be used at the beginning or end of a gong therapy session.

Traditional Kundalini Mantras

Here are three Kundalini mantras that support healing and transformation:

Ra Ma Da Sa
Sa Say So Hung

This mantra works on balancing the elements (fire, water, earth and air) and brings the energy of the infinite into the finite form.

Guru Guru Wahe Guru
Guru Ram Das Guru

Said to create miracles in healing, this mantra also brings the practitioner into the neutrality of the heart center.

Wahe Guru (pronounced Wah-hey Guroo)

This simple sound is a trikuti mantra that blends the three *gunas*, or aspects of creation (sattva, rajas, and tamas), into one form.

Ayurvedic Single-Sound Mantras

For clients who may not have a mantra practice, they can use the traditional single-sound seed (or *bija*) mantras used in Ayurvedic practices. These simple mantras are said to be effective in activating energy flow to different areas of the body as well as balancing the chakras. (Note that the **"A"** sound in the following bija mantras are pronounced **"Aah."**)

MANTRA	BENEFITS	CHAKRA
LAM	• Increases joy, grace, grounding, security. • Balances Kapha and reduces stress • Aids skeletal structure, colon, and excretory systems, adrenal glands	FIRST (Root)
VAM	• Increases flow, change, creativity, spontaneity • Balances Kapha, improves relationships • Affects left side of body • Aids lower abdomen, kidneys, pancreas and reproductive system	SECOND (Sacral)
RAM	• Increases willpower, energy, confidence • Balances Pitta and improves self-esteem • Affects right side of body • Aids legs, liver, intestine, digestive system	THIRD (Navel)
YAM	• Increases movement, compassion, neutrality • Balances Vata, strengthens immune system • Aids circulatory system, arms, hands, and heart	FOURTH (Heart)
HAM	• Increases receptivity, release, identity • Balance Vata, improves communication • Aids head, lungs, and respiratory system	FIFTH (Throat)
KSHAM	• Increases perception and intuition • Aids mind and mental abilities	SIXTH (Brow)
OM	• Increases connectivity and divinity • Aids emotional and spiritual balance	SEVENTH (Crown)

Affirmations

In yoga there is the practice of creating a *Sankalpa*, or a resolution that forms in the heart to guide us in our life. In the Western world, we can call this a positive affirmation or an intention.

Affirmations, or sankalpas, are phrased in the present tense and in an affirmative manner that connects the user of the affirmation to a desired or definite outcome. Some examples are: "I am healed in every cell of my body," or "I am happy in the present moment," or simply "I am good."

During the gong therapy session, and before the gong is played, the client can be asked to allow a positive intention or personal affirmation to arise in the consciousness in that moment, and silently repeat it three times. At the end of the session, the client is asked to repeat the original affirmation three times again. Following the session, the affirmation or *sankalpa* can be used at the beginning or end of each day over the next several days or weeks.

The therapist can also suggest positive healing affirmations based upon a client's particular need or condition that the session is working on. For example, the following table suggests five affirmations for each chakra. The client can repeat one or all five of these affirmations, depending upon the chakra being addressed during the session. Alternatively, any of these affirmations in the following table can be selected for the client to practice regardless if a specific chakra is being worked with or not.

CHAKRA	AFFIRMATIONS
FIRST Root Chakra	I am safe. I am secure. I am grounded. I am prosperous. I am here.
SECOND Sacral Chakra	I am connected. I am spontaneous. I am worthy. I am creative. I am deserving.
THIRD Navel Chakra	I am able. I am strong. I am willful. I am self-sufficient. I am determined.
FOURTH Heart Chakra	I am compassionate. I am neutral. I am willing. I am balanced. I am accepting.
FIFTH Throat Chakra	I am truthful. I am clear. I am effective. I am receptive. I am expressive.
SIXTH Third Eye Chakra	I am perceptive. I am intuitive. I am focused. I am guided. I am ready.
SEVENTH Crown Chakra	I am aware. I am trusting. I am divine. I am aligned. I am One.

Beyond the Gong: Using Other Therapeutic Sounds

Along with mantras and affirmations, other sacred healing sounds may be used during the gong therapy session. The therapist may chant, pray, or sing during the session if that is part of their healing tradition or if the client is open and prepared for the experience.

Mantras and sacred songs can be played while the gong is being played, allowing the recorded sound and music to intertwine and support the gong at either an audible or sub-audible level.

If the gong therapist is skilled in other sound healing modalities, such as singing bowls, drums, flutes, tuning forks, and similar instruments, then these may also be used, if they can be skillfully juxtapose before or after the gong playing session. In any case, care should be taken that not too many sounds are introduced or that the gong is subordinated as the primary healing instrument.

Remember that the Gong itself is the Mother of all mantras, sounds and music.

Yoga Nidra: Relaxation and Guided Meditation

The techniques of deep relaxation, guided meditation and visualization can be combined into a powerful healing experience called Yoga Nidra, or "yogic sleep." When used with the sound of the gong during a therapy session, Yoga Nidra can heighten awareness, enable self-understanding, integrate transformational changes and accelerate the healing process.

Using Yoga Nidra in a gong therapy session can be as simple as using basic guided relaxation techniques by directing awareness to different areas of the body, or it can be a visualization meditation used either before, during or after the gong is played.

Examples of Yoga Nidra sessions can be found in various books on the subject, including my book, *Teaching Gong Yoga*. The following structure may be used to develop your own guided relaxation and meditation scripts.

Structure of a Yoga Nidra Relaxation Session

Setting an Intention – At the beginning of Yoga Nidra relaxation, the client should select a precise, clear and positive intention or resolve for the session, such as "I experience radiant health," or "I am free of all pain." This intention may be repeated silently three times by the client.

Awareness of Body – While in a state of relaxation after setting the intention, the participant's awareness is systematically directed to the different parts of the body. By rotating the awareness through all areas of the body in an automatic and spontaneous fashion, a body-mind state is created that begins the process of integration. Generally, a specific sequence is used to direct body awareness, beginning with the right hand, the right side, moving to the left side, to the back of the body, to the front of the body, the head, face, and back down to the legs.

Awareness of Breath – After the rotation of consciousness, an awareness of the breath is established, either through counting or breathing into different areas or points on the body. This awakens the flow of prana and energy to every cell in the body.

Awareness of Feelings and Sensations – Now feelings and emotions are awakened, experienced, and removed through a directed focusing on pairs of opposites, such as hot and cold, joy and sadness, love and fear, light and dark. This contrasting of opposites through words or imagery allows for emotional balancing and relaxation and integration of the brain hemispheres.

Guided Visualization - The last stage of Yoga Nidra involves visualizations by the participant based upon suggestions from the instructor. This is the time to implement the sample meditation scripts in this section, or feel free to use other guided meditation or relaxation sequences that you develop on your own.

Guided Relaxation and Visualization for the Chakras

This guided visualization and relaxation can be used to help the client or therapist determine the energy center or chakra that may need attention during the gong playing session. When you complete the guided relaxation, allow the client to share what you what they discovered during their journey and use that information to determine how you will play the gong. You may also choose to play the gong during the visualization and relaxation as part of the session.

Read the following the script and modify in your own words.

Relax the body and begin to deepen the breath. Feel the rise and fall of the diaphragm as you lengthen and slow the breath.

Now breathe in from the soles of the feet to the crown of the head. Let the breath flow from the feet all the way up to the crown of the head as you inhale. As you exhale, feel the breath flow down from the crown of the head to the soles of the feet. Feeling the breath move through the entire body as you inhale and as you exhale.

(Pause while the client continues with the breath)

Now bring your breath and your attention to the base of the body at the tip of the spine. Breathe fully into that area, around the base of the spine, and simply notice any energy or feelings in that area of the body. Breathe in and out at the base of the spine.
(Pause)

Feel the energy at the base of the spine. Does it feel open or closed? Heavy or light? Is there a feeling or emotion associated with this area? Is there a color or an image that comes to mind? Focus at the base of the spine and simply be aware of what you are sensing and feeling. Consciously breathe in and out of this area and then let your breath and awareness relax.
(Pause)

Now allow your awareness to move up to the area behind the pubic bone and the pelvic area. Breathe into the hips and the reproductive area. Breathe fully into the area around the pelvis, and simply notice any energy or feelings in that area of the body. Breathe in and out the pelvic area.

(Pause)

Feel the energy at the pelvic area. Does it feel open or closed? Heavy or light? Is there a feeling or emotion associated with this area? Is there a color or an image that comes to mind? Focus on the pelvic area and simply be aware of what you are sensing and feeling. Consciously breathe in and out of this area and then let your breath and awareness relax.

(Pause)

Now allow your awareness to move up to the solar plexus, the area between the navel and the ribs, and begin to explore that area, noticing the feeling and sensations within that center. Notice the response as you take the breath into it, feeling all the way from the solar plexus to the back to the spine.

(Pause)

Feel the energy around the solar plexus. Does it feel open or closed? Heavy or light? Is there a feeling or emotion associated with this area? Is there a color or an image that comes to mind? Focus on the solar plexus area and simply be aware of what you are sensing and feeling. Consciously breathe in and out of this area and then let your breath and awareness relax.

(Pause)

Then bring your awareness up to the heart center noticing the place where the energy feels strongest in the center of the chest and begin to explore that energy center by taking the breath through it. Notice how that center responds to the breath; whether it begins to open out or feels closed in; if it feels clear or if there is a sense of layers covering the heart center.

(Pause)

Feel the energy around the heart. Does it feel open or closed? Heavy or light? Is there a feeling or emotion associated with this area? Is there a color or an image that comes to mind? Focus on the heart area and simply be aware of what you are sensing and feeling. Consciously breathe in and out of this area and then let your breath and awareness relax.

(Pause)

Now allow your awareness to move up to throat and the neck, and begin to explore that area, noticing the feeling and sensations within that energy center of the body. Notice the response as you take the breath into the throat, feeling the breath entering and moving in and out of the throat.

(Pause)

Feel the energy around the throat. Does it feel open or closed? Heavy or light? Is there a feeling or emotion associated with this area? Is there a color or an image that comes to mind? Focus on the throat area and simply be aware of what you are sensing and feeling. Consciously breathe in and out of this area and then let your breath and awareness relax.

(Pause)

Now allow your awareness to come up to a place between the eyebrows and feel the energy itself guiding you back between the eyebrows. Notice if you can sense being drawn inward or perhaps a sense that the door is opening to a place without time or description. Look inward and feel any sensations or experience any colors that may be associated with the third eye energy center. See if there is a vision or an image that presents itself here.

(Pause)

Focus on the third eye area and simply be aware of what you are sensing and feeling. Consciously breathe in and out of this area and then let your breath and awareness relax.

(Pause)

Now bring your awareness to the top of the head, the crown chakra, and visualize the area right above the head. Sense any opening around the crown of the head or any energy coming into the head. What are the sensations, the images and the color that may be associated with this energy center.

(Pause)

Focus on the crown of the head and simply be aware of what you are sensing and feeling. Consciously breathe in and out of this area and then let your breath and awareness relax.

(Pause)

Please inhale deeply and then exhale slowly and completely. Completely relax and now allow the sound of the gong to go to the area of the body that you feel needs the most healing energy and attention. Let your awareness rest there and let this sound fill this area with healing light and energy. Fill this area with healing light and the sound of the Gong.

(Pause)

Begin playing the gong.

Healing Light Yoga Nidra

Begin by having the client relax and use the following script. If you wish, you can play the gong softly as you read the script, or wait until the guided meditation is finished before you play the gong.

Read the following the script and modify in your own words:

Relax the folded hands over the heart.

Inhale through the nose and exhale slowly through pursed lips.

Inhale through the nose and exhale slowly through pursed lips.

Inhale through the nose and exhale slowly through pursed lips.

Inhale through the nose and exhale slowly through pursed lips.

Inhale through the nose and exhale slowly through pursed lips.

Let the breath relax. Let the hands relax.

(Pause)

Listen and visualize each image that I describe. Feel the sensations around each image. Then let your mind move immediately to the next image.

(Pause)
(After each image is repeated twice, pause briefly.)

Melting ice in a stream ... Melting ice in a stream

Bird singing in the night ... Bird singing in the night

Dying embers in a fire ... Dying embers in a fire

Baby laughing ... Baby laughing

Old man crying ... Old man crying

Dog rolling in the snow ... Dog rolling in the snow

Buddha smiling ... Buddha smiling

Flowers dying ... Flowers dying

Starless sky ... Starless sky

Holding hands ... Holding hands

Endless night ... Endless night

Cat on a bed ... Cat on a bed

Sunlight on a table ... sunlight on a table

Cross of gold ... Cross of gold

Mother nursing child ... Mother nursing child

Cold wet earth ... Cold wet earth

Relaxing in a warm bath ... Relaxing in a warm bath

(Long Pause)

Now feel the beat of your heart, feel the beat of your heart.
Let the breath fill you. Breathe out and let the breath leave you.
Let the breath fill you. Breathe out and let the breath leave you.
Hear the sound of your breath. Hear the sound of your breath.
Feel the stillness within you. Feel the stillness within you.

(Long Pause)

Now visualize yourself standing alone in a snowy meadow on a dark winter night.

See yourself standing in a snowy meadow on a winter night.

Feel the cold air on your face. Feel the cold air on your face.

Walk across the empty meadow. Feel the night around you. Feel the snow beneath you. Feel the cool air on your face.

Walk to the end of the meadow. Walk to the end of the meadow.

See a hill in front of you. See a hill in front of you.

Begin to walk up the hill. Begin to walk up the hill.

Feel the coolness of the winter night. Feel the coolness of night.

Come to the top of the hill. Come to the top of the hill.

Sit and relax on top of the hill. Sit and relax on top of the hill.

Sitting in the night, sitting in the night. Feel the wind on your face.

Endless night, endless night.

Moonless night, moonless night.

See a ray of light. See a ray of light in the night.

See the light. See the light.

Ending night, ending night.

Light returning, light returning.

Sunrise coming, sunrise coming.

Sunlight bright, sunlight bright.

Feel the light on your face, feel the light on your face.

Feel the light inside, feel the light inside.

Sun-filled heart, sun-filled heart.

Feel the light, feel the light.

Feel the light inside, feel the light inside.

Sunlight bright, sunlight bright.

Feel the light around you, feel the light around you.

Be the light, be the light.

Be the light, be the light.

Be the light, be the light.

(Pause)

Begin playing the gong.

Point-to-Point Deep Relaxation

Let the client relax and connect to the breath as the diaphragm rises and falls. Use the following script and remember to pause at the end of each instruction to allow for time for the full inhale and exhale. If you wish, you can play the gong softly with a single downward strike each time the breath is exhaled.

Read the following script and modify in your own words:

1) Inhale the breath slowly up from the **bottom of the feet** to the **crown of the head.**
2) Exhale down from the **crown of the head** to the **bottom of the feet.**

---

3) Inhale the breath slowly up from the **bottom of the feet** to the **crown of the head.**
4) Exhale slowly down from the **crown of the head** to the **ankles.**

---

5) Inhale the breath slowly up from the **ankles** to the **crown of the head.**
6) Exhale slowly down from the **crown of the head** to the **ankles.**

---

7) Inhale the breath slowly up from the **ankles** to the **crown of the head.**
8) Exhale slowly down from the **crown of the head** to the **knees.**

---

9) Inhale the breath slowly up from the **knees** to the **crown of the head.**
10) Exhale slowly down from the **crown of the head** to the **knees.**

---

11) Inhale the breath slowly up from the **knees** to the **crown of the head.**
12) Exhale slowly down from the **crown of the head** to the **base of the spine.**

---

13) Inhale the breath slowly up from the **base of the spine** to the **crown of the head.**
14) Exhale slowly down from the **crown of the head** to the **base of the spine.**

16) Inhale the breath slowly up from the **base of the spine** to the **crown of the head**.

17) Exhale slowly down from the **crown of the head** to the **navel point**.

18) Inhale the breath up from the **navel point** to the **crown of the head**.

19) Exhale slowly down from the **crown of the head** to the **navel point**.

20) Inhale the breath up from the **navel point** to the **crown of the head**.

21) Exhale slowly down from the **crown of the head** to the **heart center**.

22) Inhale the breath slowly up from the **heart center** to the **crown of the head**.

23) Exhale slowly down from the **crown of the head** to the **heart center**.

24) Inhale the breath up from the **heart center** to the **crown of the head**.

25) Exhale slowly down from the **crown of the head** to the **throat**.

26) Inhale the breath slowly up from the **throat** to the **crown of the head**.

27) Exhale slowly down from the **crown of the head** to the **throat**.

28) Inhale the breath slowly up from the **throat** to the **crown of the head**.

29) Exhale slowly down from the **crown of the head** to the **third eye**.

30) Inhale the breath slowly up from the **third eye** to the **crown of the head**.

31) Exhale slowly down from the **crown of the head** to the **third eye**.

32) Inhale the breath slowly up from the **third eye** to the **crown of the head**.

33) Exhale slowly down from the **crown of the head** to the **third eye**.

34) Inhale the breath slowly up from the **third eye** to the **crown of the head**.

35) Exhale slowly down from the **crown of the head** to the **throat**.

36) Inhale the breath slowly up from the **throat** to the **crown of the head**.

37) Exhale slowly down from the **crown of the head** to the **heart**.

---

38) Inhale the breath slowly up from the **heart center** to the **crown of the head**.

39) Exhale slowly down from the **crown of the head** to the **navel point**.

---

40) Inhale the breath slowly up from the **navel point** to the **crown of the head**.

41) Exhale slowly down from the **crown of the head** to the **base of the spine**.

---

42) Inhale the breath slowly up from the **base of the spine** to the **crown of the head**.

43) Exhale slowly down from the **crown of the head** to the **knees**.

---

44) Inhale the breath slowly up from the **knees** to the **crown of the head**.

45) Exhale slowly down from the **crown of the head** to the **ankles**.

---

46) Inhale the breath slowly up from the **ankles** to the **crown of the head**.

47) Exhale down from the **crown of the head** to the **bottom of the feet**.

---

48) Inhale the breath slowly up from the **bottom of the feet** to the **crown of the head**.

49) Exhale down from the **crown of the head** to the **bottom of the feet**.

---

50) Inhale the breath slowly up from the **bottom of the feet** to the **crown of the head**.

51) Exhale down from the **crown of the head** to the **bottom of the feet**.

Relax the breath. Let the breath relax. Relax deeply. Relax deeply. Relax into the sound of the gong.

Begin playing the gong.

Point to Point Breathing

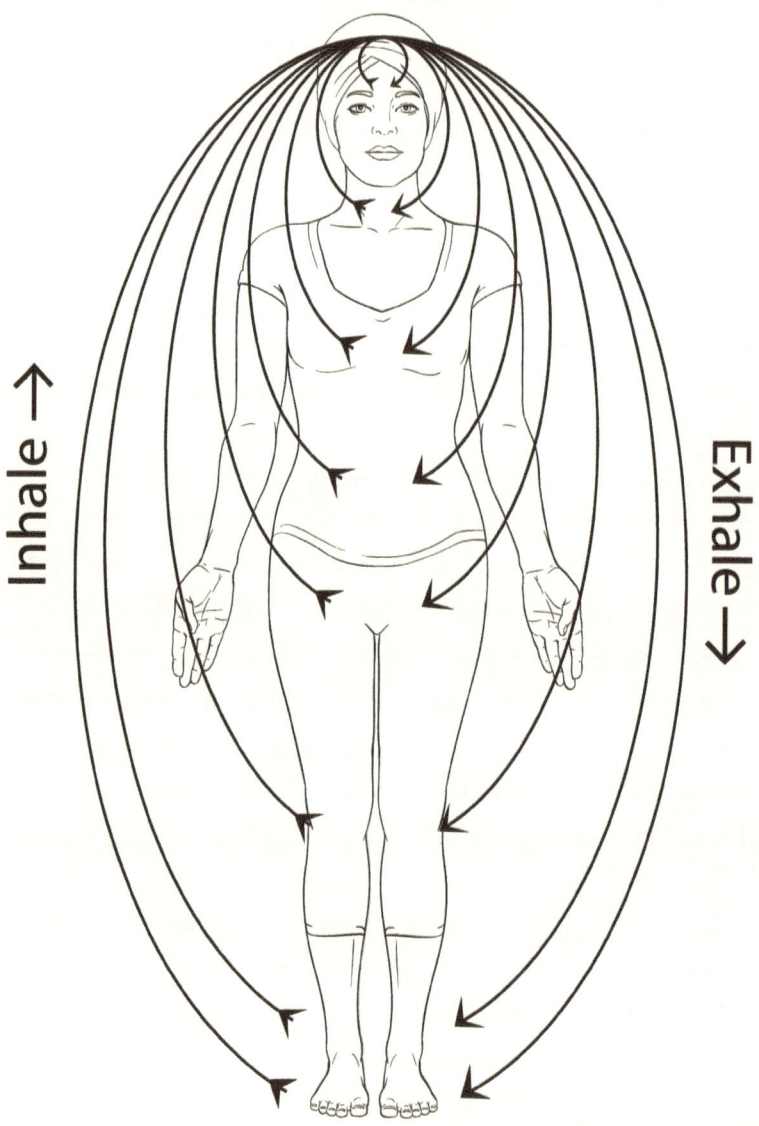

Gongs for Therapy

The gong is both the instrument and the energetic extension of the therapist. As such, its importance cannot be overstated. It is through the gong that the therapist's innate healing abilities and prana are transferred, and over time the boundaries between the gong and the gong player merge into a healing entity that is beyond flesh and metal.

Your success as a gong therapist depends upon three things: 1) Your playing skills and techniques, 2) Your daily spiritual practice (sadhana), and 3) Your gong.

The gong becomes the projection of the therapist's intuitive connection to the client, another voice, another pair of hands, and another heartbeat that is felt on an exceedingly intimate level by the the client. As such, a gong used for therapy is more than a musical instrument; it is sacred medicine and an agent of the divine.

Fortunately, we live in a time when some of the best gongs ever made are available to anyone with comparatively modest resources. In ancient times, gongs were only played by very few, usually a privileged priestly class, and truly excellent gongs were scarce and prohibitively expensive until the later twentieth century.

Today there are artisans creating handmade gongs, as well as several respected commercial manufacturers producing high quality instruments. We have more gongs to choose from today than ever before in history, and it can be overwhelming to the beginning therapist. Other than personally playing the gongs, your best guidance for a therapy gong will come from other gong therapists and players (although realize they too have their own biases and filters).

There are basic guidelines and practical suggestions, however, for selecting the gongs and the basic equipment you need to practice gong therapy, and that is the purpose of this chapter. Let's start with the equipment and then examine the types of gongs best suitable for therapy.

Selecting the Gong Stand

The stand is an important consideration for a gong therapist as it will influence your style of playing, inform your therapy environment and affect the experience of your clients.

When selecting a stand, here are the guidelines and options:

1) Size of the Gong
2) Playing seated or playing standing
3) Stationary or mobile stand
4) Number of gongs

Size of the Stand

Gongs are sized by diameter and usually range from 20 inches (50 centimeters) to 80 inches (2 meters). Some stands are fixed in size which means a stand made for a 24-inch gong will only hold that size or smaller. Some stands can hold a range of sizes, from a 2-inch difference in the size of the gongs to as much as an 8-inch difference. There are also adjustable stands that can hold gongs of all sizes up to 40 inches. The extra-large stands required for gongs larger than 40 inches are rarely, if ever, used in individual gong therapy sessions.

If you have a dedicated stand for each gong, then you can use a fixed size stand. If you anticipate adding different size gongs, you may want to select a stand that accepts a wider size range of gongs or the special stands that can hold almost any size gong. Stands are relatively inexpensive compared to gongs, so buy the one you are most comfortable with and consider how you may expand if you use multiple or larger gongs later.

Seated or Standing

Gongs are played in a seated (or kneeling) position or in a standing position, and there are stands for seated players and standing players, as well those that are adjustable for both playing styles.

There are advantages and challenges with either playing position. Do experiment with both styles if you have only played in one position.

However, you will ultimately be influenced in your selection of a stand by how you structure your gong therapy environment. If you plan on using a massage or therapy table for your client, you will choose stands that permit the gongs to be positioned near the level of the table. If the client will be on the floor, you will be better served by having a floor stand that you can play while seated. Also consider if you will need to move your stands from location to location as that will be a factor as well.

Finally, you may consider an adjustable height stand that can be raised or lowered for therapy situations, or simply have different stands for both seated playing sessions and standing playing sessions.

Stationary or Mobile Stand

Some gong stands may be fitted with wheels that lock and unlock, allowing the stand to be easily moved during a therapy session should you wish to change playing positions in relation to the client. If you have enough stationary stands for your gongs, then the mobile stands are not necessary. However, if you find yourself using multiple gongs, you may want to be able to roll the stands in and out rather than moving gongs from stand to stand.

Number of Gongs

Some gong stands can be adjusted to hold either one or two gongs. These double stands can be adjusted so you can play the lower gong while sitting on the floor and the upper gong while standing up, adding to the flexibility of how you arrange your gongs.

Selecting the Mallets

There are soft covered mallets, there are hard yarn mallets, there are rubber ball or "rubbing" mallets, and there are mallets too small and mallets too large! Typically, mallets are often suggested for the size and type of gong you play, although you may want to use a mallet one size down from the manufacturer's recommended size.

Smaller mallets give more control over volume since you will typically play softer in therapy session with the gong positioned close to the client. However, you will need a full size mallet to pull the rich and deep fundamental healing tones from your gong.

Fortunately, you are not limited to one mallet. In fact, if you are playing therapeutically, you will likely have a collection of mallets to produce different sounds. And if you are playing multiple gongs on different stands, you can dedicate mallets to each stand to get the best sound from each gong.

At the minimum, you will want two mallets, with one mallet smaller than the other, so you can vary the volume and striking areas.

The specialty mallets, such as the round rubbing balls that create the arching overtones, can be fun if not over used. Watch the tendency, however, to load up on too many mallets. You may end up distracting yourself or your client with all your equipment choices.

Therapeutic Gongs

First, all gongs are therapeutic. Second, some are more therapeutic than others!

Selecting a therapy gong is the most personal choice you make as a gong therapist. The gong will become an extension of yourself, your healing energy, and your heart. You will touch and heal through the gong. In many ways, it is the most intimate intermediary you will have in a healing relationship.

Often the gong may select you, either by destiny, circumstance or divine guidance. You can listen to the gongs, live or on-line, but you only get a good feel for the sound when you play it yourself. Most people rarely get to try out the gongs before they buy them so it is important to buy a recognized or respected brand, or from a recommended artisan.

There are guidelines, however, you can use when buying your first (or tenth!) therapeutic gong.

Sizes of Gongs

Size is a major consideration in selecting a gong, but that does not mean that the bigger the gong, the better the gong is for therapy. Indeed, since the gongs used in therapy sessions are played closer to the listener than in most other environments, small gongs can give excellent results.

In general, gongs that range from 24 inches to 32 inches (60 to 80 centimeters) are excellent for therapeutic work. They are large enough to produce a full sound yet do not overwhelm. While the larger gongs in the 34 inches to 40 inches range (85 to 95 centimeters) are amazing agents of transformation, they need to be played judiciously in the smaller and more intimate therapeutic settings.

If you have a small therapeutic gong, get a larger one next time – you will discover that even a 2-inch difference in size can be profoundly different in effect. If you have a large gong, get a smaller one next time, and notice the way it subtly changes your playing. The contrast in the sound quality with the various sizes can allow you to discover the gong ensemble that serves your playing style best.

Eastern Gongs Versus Western Gongs

Another way to categorize the gongs is by the place of origin. Almost all gongs are Oriental or European made. While this category seems somewhat geographically arbitrary, there are true distinctions even among the great variety being offered from each region.

There is a different philosophy and approach in the Eastern and Western gong making. The range of Eastern gongs is breathtaking; however most Western gong players have an overwhelming preference for Western made gongs. While some Western gong therapists do include an Oriental-made gong (particularly the large-size Chinese wind gongs that produce such a unique sound) in their repertoire, it is the European manufactured gongs that make up the great majority of gongs used for therapy in the Western world.

One theory advanced for the preference for the Western gongs over the Eastern gongs is the fundamental differences in the manufacturing process.

The Eastern approach to gong making is a hot forging process that casts the metal. The forging process dampens the soft and amorphous crystalline structure of the cast bronze that creates an inner dampening factor. The sound quality of the metal is limited and there are fewer resiliencies in the surface of the gong so the overtones become muted. This does create a single deep consolidated sound but somewhat lacking in versatility. Having said that, there is definitely a place in therapy work for that deep tone that comes from a forged gong.

In the West, the gongs are not forged but are hammered from cold rolled sheet metal that has a small amount of nickel silver to give higher frequencies and greater brilliance of sound. The thin sheet of hammered bronze, as opposed to the usually thicker Eastern gongs, impart an elasticity and rebound on the gong strike that produces the complex carrying sound and overtones that enhance the therapeutic nature of the sound.

Categories of Gongs

Within the world of Western gongs, there are two major categories: (1) Gongs that are tuned to a specific frequency, and (2) Gongs that have a variable frequency, or non-tuned gongs.

Tuned gongs, as their name suggests, are tuned to a specific frequency distinguished by such designations as "D#-151.27 Hz" or "B1-126.27 Hz." Common brand name examples of Western tuned gongs are the Paiste and Meinl Planetary Gongs (tuned to the orbital frequencies of the planets) or the Meinl Symphonic Gongs that are tuned to a specific half-tone range such as "A#1-B1" or "E2-F2."

Variable Frequency or Non-Tuned gongs have a versatile harmonic sound structure that create complex overtones and are exceedingly versatile in the sounds they can produce. The more recognizable Western brands of the non-tuned gongs are the Paiste Symphonic Gongs (symphonic in the true sense of the word of "uniting sounds into harmony") and the Paiste Sound Creation Gongs that create a wide range of sound colors and resonant blending.

Tuned Versus Non-Tuned Gongs for Therapy

Both types of gongs play an important role in Gong Therapy. The non-tuned gongs are the great generalists. They have a wide range of applications and are exceptionally versatile in their approach and execution. The tuned gongs are expert specialists, able to reach deep within to effect a decided outcome. Both types of gongs play well together.

The non-tuned gongs are fundamental to the practice of gong therapy. If you can only have one gong, the non-tuned gong with its wide range of sound and expression can be adapted to most circumstances and needs. The size is the significant difference in the effects the non-tuined gongs produce, and the 26" (66 cm), 28" (71 cm), 30" (76 cm), and 32" (81 cm) are all excellent entry-level gongs. Every therapist should have one of these.

The tuned gongs are the special tools of the therapist. It does take some experience and skill to work with the tuned gongs, not because they are difficult to play, but because of the subtlety and sophistication of their effects. While you may go through life with only one excellent non-tuned gong appropriately sized, you will soon discover that you can never have too many tuned gongs. They are tools for the specialist, and each one has its own unique therapeutic effects.

Usually a gong tuned to a specific frequency comes in one size, ranging from 24" to 38", depending upon the gong. For example, if you want a gong tuned to the orbital frequency of Mercury (141.27 Hz), your only size choice is 32 inches. In other words, tuned gongs are selected by frequency and not by size. While you can investigate the therapeutic effects of each frequency as you consider which tuned gong to get, the experience you and your clients will be the deciding factor in their degree of success.

However, you may find the following table of frequencies helpful as you investigate the relationship between the tuned frequencies of various gongs and the chakras they affect. For a guide, the Paiste Planetary gong that is tuned to the given frequency for each chakra is specified in the table.

Chakra	Frequency	Paiste Planetary Gong
First (Root)	194.18 Hz	Sidereal Day (194.71 Hz)
Second (Sacral)	210.42 Hz	Synodic Moon (210.42 Hz)
Third (Solar Plexus)	126.22 Hz	Sun (126.27 Hz)
Fourth (Heart)	136.10 Hz	Earth (136.10 Hz)
Fifth (Throat)	141.27 Hz	Mercury (141.27 Hz)
Sixth (Third Eye)	221.23 Hz	Venus (221.23 Hz)
Seventh (Crown)	172.06 Hz	Platonic Year (172.06 Hz)

While tuned gongs can be helpful in working with the frequencies of specific chakras, any gong well-played can work on all the chakra frequencies, regardless of its tuning.

How Many Gongs?

You can practice gong therapy very effectively with only one gong. Theoretically, you could have dozens of gongs, in every size and frequency, but this would require a high level of expertise and developed intuition to understand how to use them in any reasonable way, and more than likely, you would likely fixate on your favorite six or seven gongs anyway.

Realistically, it is hard to imagine why you would ever need to use more than eight gongs during a therapy session. This would require that you have a double gong stand on each side of the client, as well as a highly developed degree of technical sophistication to know how to use them all effectively and not be a distraction to yourself of your client.

For most sessions, one to four gongs will suffice very well. Having too many gongs during a session can disorient the client as they try to identify or anticipate all the different gongs you may use, which can shift their focus away from their own experience.

Gong is not a drum

Or a musical instrument;

Gong is God.

Yogi Bhajan

Gong Playing Techniques for Therapy

Gongs have been played throughout ages and cultures for many purposes. Gongs have been played in rituals for marriages and deaths, in ceremonies for initiation and coronation, in orchestras for Western symphonies and Eastern theater, in yoga classes for relaxation and meditation, at social functions and cultural events, and at outdoor festivals and tribal gatherings.

They have been played in emergencies and war to alert the populace and in entertainment and spectacles to entrance the audience. Gongs have been played by shamans, priests, rock stars, and even sales managers to celebrate a transaction.

In all these occasions, there was a specific purpose in which the gong was played. And so it is also true in Gong Therapy. There is a specific way to play the gong that makes it therapeutic for both the player and the client.

Characteristics of Playing the Gong for Therapy

The primary characteristic of playing the gong for therapy is that it is played with the intention of creating a desired effect according to the needs of the individual. You are playing for an audience of one person. You are playing to relieve suffering and elevate the individual in that present moment.

As such, therapeutic gong playing is completely personal in purpose yet impersonal in nature. You will never play the same way twice for your clients. The playing is completely in the moment, with an intuitive intunement to the continually shifting needs of the client as the sound is experienced and the energy shifts.

This ability to play in the present and in response to the process that is unfolding means that it is impossible to plan how you will play in a gong therapy session. Consequently, you will need to learn the fundamentals for playing the gong for certain conditions, as well as techniques used by therapists, but ultimately you need to **rely on your intuition as you follow these guidelines** and implement these techniques. In the final sense, you cannot learn to play the gong therapeutically. You can only recognize it when you do so.

With these caveats in mind, let's look at general guidelines and examples to help you on your journey to playing therapeutically.

The Three Basic Components of Gong Playing

Whether you are playing the gong for relaxation, meditation, artistic expression or therapeutic healing, there are only three components to consider when playing:

1) Playing Area – where do you strike the gong?

2) Rhythm – how fast or slow do you strike the gong?

3) Volume – how soft or hard do you strike the gong?

The effects created by the gong player depends upon how these three components are implemented and varied through recurring sequences of patterns and contrasts.

The basis of therapeutic gong playing consists of varying one or two of these components while keeping the third component constant. For example, playing the same area of the gong at the same volume level but varying the rhythm from fast to slow and then slow to fast; or keeping the rhythm constant but varying both the volume and the area of the gong that is being played.

These three playing methods (rhythm, volume and playing area) create eight combinations of playing possibilities:

Rhythm	Volume	Playing Area	Energetic Effects
Constant	Constant	Varies	Balances energy
Constant	Varies	Varies	Moves energy
Constant	Varies	Constant	Sedates energy
Varies	Varies	Constant	Raises energy
Varies	Constant	Constant	Balances energy
Varies	Constant	Varies	Moves energy
Constant	Constant	Constant	Consolidates energy
Varies	Varies	Varies	Disperses energy

Gong therapists typically use three or more of these combinations in a therapy session. Now let's look how the playing areas, the rhythm and the volume create different therapeutic effects.

The Gong Playing Areas

The surface of the gong may be divided into three striking areas: Center area, Mid-area, and Rim area. On some gongs, you can see these areas clearly delimited by the finish on the surface. The center area appears to be like a small sun with a diameter about one-quarter the size of the entire gong. The rim area is slightly rough and extends a few inches around the edge. The mid-area between the rim and the center is the largest playing area, sometimes a color between the darker rim and the brighter center. Each playing area produces a different quality of sound when struck.

Striking the gong near the center area gives a rich, enduring and carrying sound–almost like a strong fundamental note. Striking in the mid-area between the center and rim produces a deep, complete and swelling sound–rich and complex in tone coloring. Striking in the rim area gives an airy, sparkling and roaring sound–partial tones that transcend any specific pitch. During therapeutic playing, the majority of the playing is in the mid-area, followed by the center area, and finally the rim area.

The rim area is used to release and disperse blocked energy, and so should be used sparingly in order to not dissipate the client. The rim area can create an expansion of possibilities and potentialities, however, a sense of going beyond the current limitation of self, and can be a powerful playing area during a therapy session.

The center area is used to collect and build energy, and can be effectively paired with playing the rim in order to exchange energy in and out of the body. It is an area of the gong that creates a sense of integration and being in the new self.

The mid-area balances and distributes energy. Many playing possibilities exist in this area and are discussed in the sections, Percussion Points and Gong Maps.

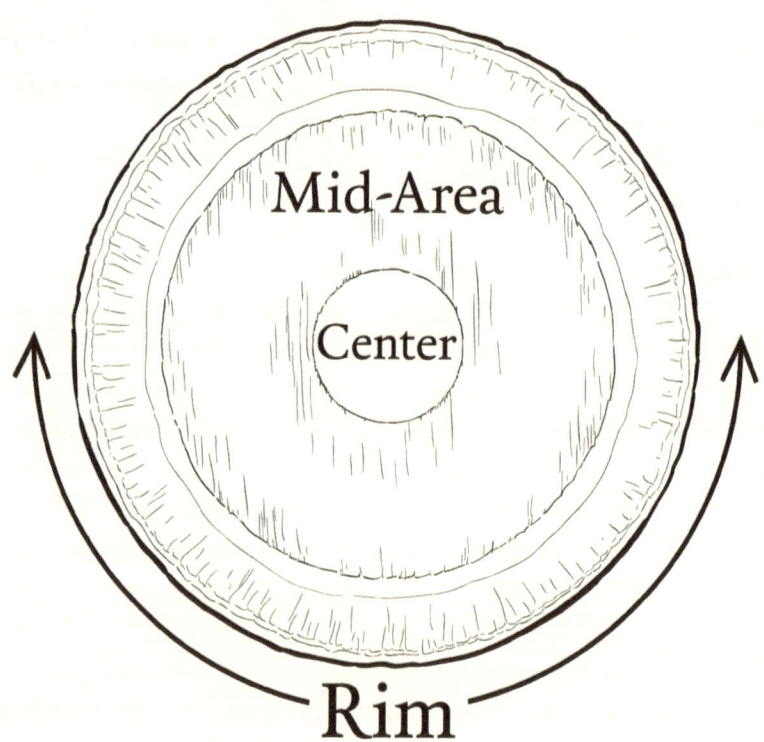

The Percussion Points

In addition to the three major areas, there are 14 discrete playing areas on the gong called percussion points. Think of the gong as a clock face divided into 12 areas, one for each hour. The 12 o'clock position is at the top of the gong (or more precisely in the top of the mid-area of the gong below the rim). The 6 o'clock position is at the bottom, again above the rim area. The other clock positions go around the outer mid-area of gong so there are 12 points or localized areas that can be struck. In the middle of the gong, there is a zero position so that the upper center area (before the mid-area begins) is known as "Up 0" and the lower center area is known as "Down 0." So we now have 14 total percussion points on the gong (including the two center "0" points) where the vast majority of the mallet strikes will occur.

Each percussion point produces a distinctive sound, and can be played in various sequences with other points to create a specific effect. For example, playing the percussion points 3, 6, 9, and 12 in repeated sequences distribute energy equally around the body.

The percussion points will be used when we discuss therapeutic playing patterns.

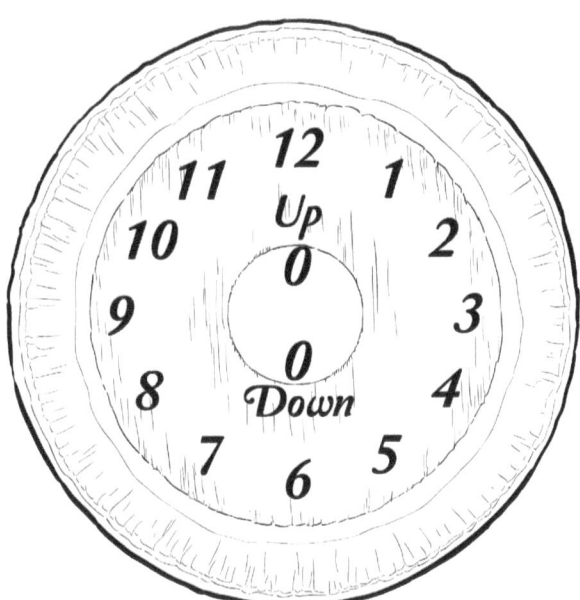

Playing Areas and Gong Maps

The concept of a gong map, that playing various areas of the gong affect different organs, glands, and body areas as well as the chakras, is based upon the concept of the Cosmic Human, or that the microcosm of the human body reflects the macrocosm of the universe. This is a common concept in yoga and medical astrology whereby the various planetary energies are contained or represented in different areas of the body, as in the case of the right side of the body is related to the Sun energy and the left side to the Moon energy. In Western philosophy, this idea of the individual containing the macrocosm is revealed in the Hermetic teachings as exemplified in the saying, "So above, so below. So within, so without."

In the case of the gong, we apply this same principle that the gong itself is also a microcosm or a representation of the human body, the energy centers of the body, and indeed all energies present in the universe. In this way, we can use the gong as an esoteric mapping method to work with these systems and energies.

Playing Areas of the Gong and the Body

The physical body and its functions can be mapped onto the gong with the top indicating the head area, the upper half of the gong corresponding to the body above the heart, the center of the gong represents the heart itself, the lower half of the gong corresponding to the body below the heart, and the bottom of the gong representing the legs and feet.

Similarly playing on the right side of the gong affects the limbs, organs, and body areas on the right, and similarly for the left side of the gong.

The following illustration shows how the body's organs and physiological systems can be associated with different playing areas of the gong as follows:

- **Area One** – Brain, pineal and pituitary glands, eyes, nose, ears, mouth, head, nervous system.

- **Area Two** – Throat, thyroid and parathyroid glands, lungs, respiratory system.

- **Area Three** – Heart, thymus gland, arms, hands, circulatory system.

- **Area Four** – Stomach, small intestine, liver, gall bladder, spleen, pancreas, digestive system.

- **Area Five** – Colon, rectum, genitals, adrenals, kidneys, bladder, reproductive and excretory systems.

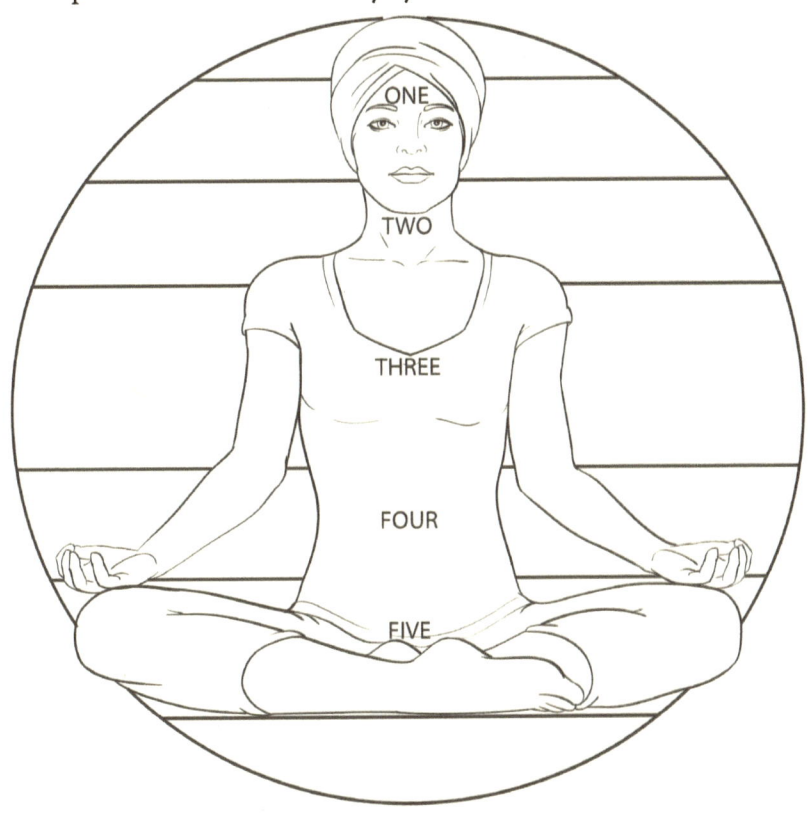

Playing Areas of the Gong and the Chakras

The area of the gong struck also affects different chakras. According to Yogi Bhajan, master of Kundalini Yoga and the gong, the seven major chakras may be accessed through the gong playing area by superimposing a map of the chakra system as it aligns up within the body, moving from bottom to top.

In this manner, the first chakra would be located at the bottom of the gong, directly above the rim area. The second chakra would be right above the first chakra and the third chakra right below the bottom center of the gong. The fourth chakra would be around the center of the gong and the fifth chakra above the top of the center of the gong. The sixth chakra is closer to the top of the gong and the seventh or crown chakra is right beneath the top rim of the gong. The aura that surrounds the energy body and the seven chakras is associated with the rim area around the gong face.

The playing areas of the gong allow the Gong therapist to access individual chakras as well as moving energy between the chakras.

Playing Areas of the Gong & the Chakras

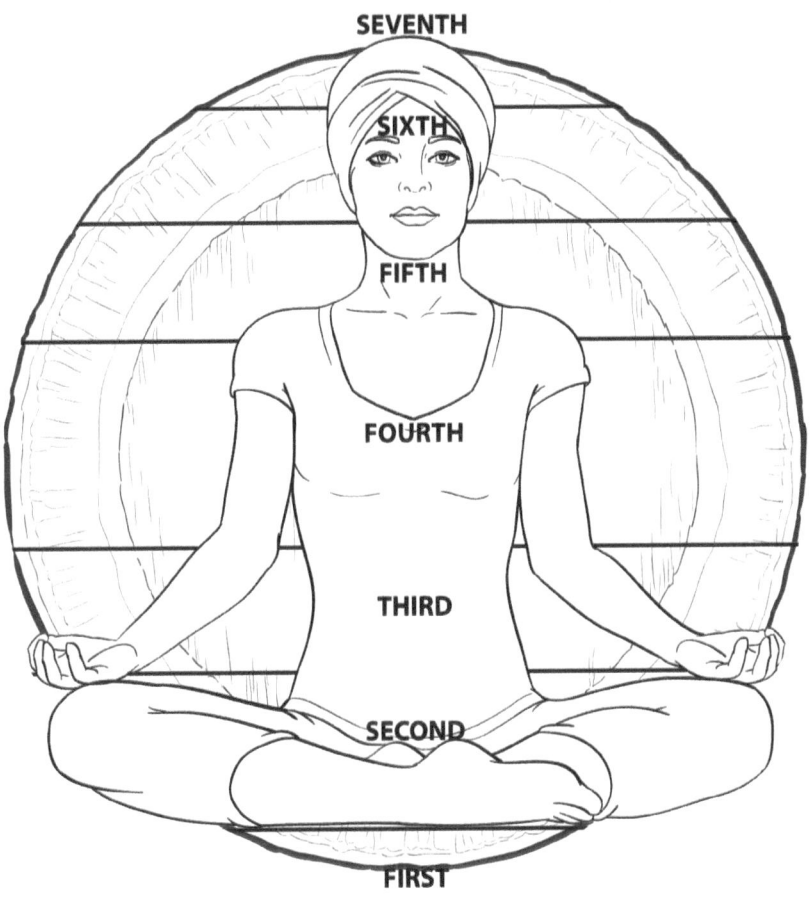

The Four Quadrants of the Gong

In addition to the playing areas for physical body and the chakras, the four quadrants of the gong (upper right, lower right, upper left and lower left) are used to produce energetic and therapeutic effects as shown in the following gong map.

Notice that the inside and outside quadrants are designated in relationship to the player. The side of the gong that corresponds to the player's dominant playing side is termed the outside half. So for right-hand players the outside half is the right side of the gong as you face it, and the left side is the outside half for left-hand players.

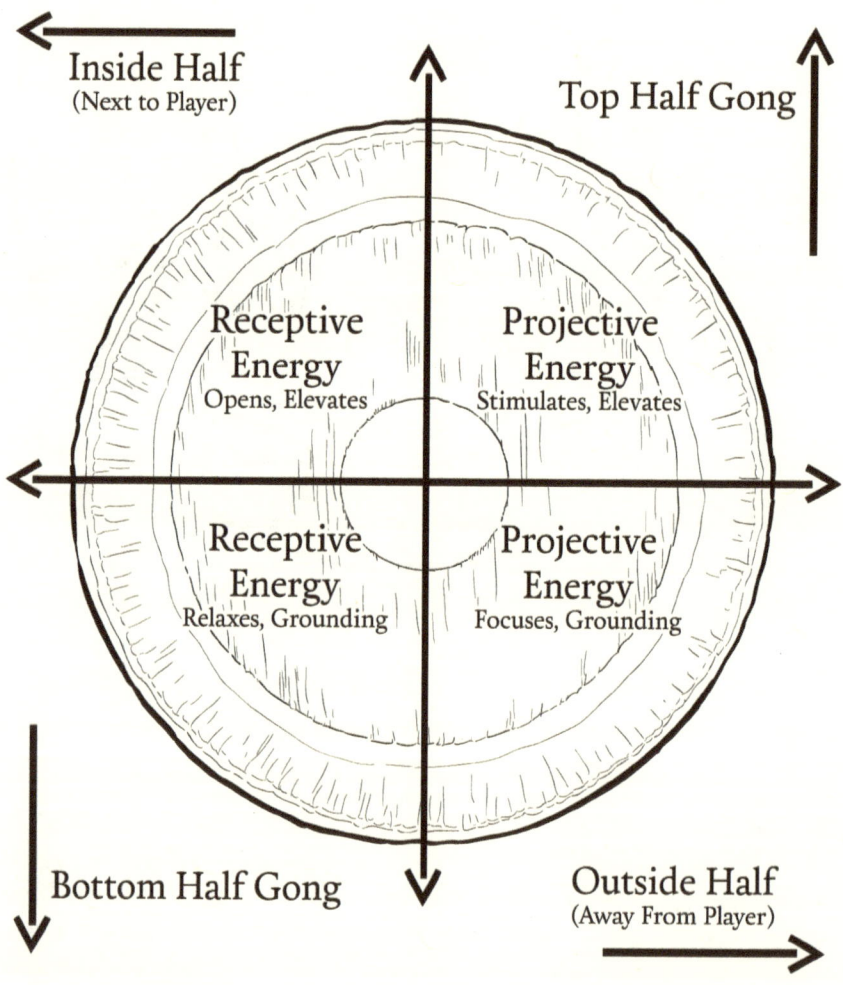

Gong Maps from a Yogi's Perspective

Through practice and intuition, the gong therapist may create their own gong maps to access and affect different areas of the body and states of mind. Yogi Bhajan, the master of the Gong and Kundalini Yoga, shared one such map he used in the early 1970s.

He divided the gong into four map areas:

1) Upper left quadrant (for left hand players, this is the upper right quadrant)

2) Lower left quadrant (for left hand players, this is the lower right quadrant)

3) The right half of the gong, top and bottom quadrants (for left hand players, this is the left half of the gong)

4) The middle area of the gong (above and below the center circle).

This gong map was used in the following playing sequence:

- Begin playing softly in the upper left quadrant (percussion points 10 and 11). This can be done for 3 minutes. This is called the "Tuning in Stage" and begins to entrance the mind.

- Begin playing more strongly into the lower left quadrant (percussion points 7 and 8). Over a span of 3 minutes, keep increasing the sound as powerful as you intuitively feel that the listener can tolerate. This is called the "Workout Stage" and helps to access and dissolve subconscious fears.

- Begin to change the playing to the right half of the gong. The sound is still strong but gradually becomes softer and more melodious, like the waves of the ocean or the voices in a choir, and is played around percussion points 1, 2, 4 and 5 over a period of 6 minutes. This is called the "Floating Stage" where there can be a disassociation with the body and mind and this is where the healing occurs.

- Finally begin to play around to the middle area of the gong (above and below the 0 percussion point) to produce the deep fundamental tones, almost like a heartbeat. The playing is steady and centering and done for 2 minutes. This is the "Integration Stage" where the body, mind and spirit coalesce into a new sense of unity through the sound of the gong.

Rhythm and Volume in Therapeutic Playing

In addition to the playing areas of the gong, the Gong therapist uses the techniques of rhythm and volume to create, cultivate, and direct the flow of energy and the attention of the client during a therapy session. Here are the basic considerations when working with rhythm and volume during a therapy session.

Fast and Slow

In general, a faster rhythm increases the movement of energy while a slower rhythm integrates the movement of energy. The faster the rhythm, the higher the chakra affected. Slow rhythms resonate with the lower chakras. Fast rhythms move energy up the chakras. Slow rhythms move energy back down the chakras. (Remember that energy needs to flow both up and down the chakras to create a balancing effect.)

The relationship between a slow rhythm and a fast rhythm is dependent upon the player's baseline, or dominant, rhythm during the session. According to a lecture by Yogi Bhajan on playing the gong, we can discern a ratio of 3:5:7 as regards slow and fast rhythm, with "5" being the baseline rhythm of the player during the session, "3" for the slow rhythm and "7" for the fast rhythm.

Using the 3:5:7 ratio, a slow rhythm is about 40% slower than the baseline rhythm, relatively speaking, and a fast rhythm is about 140% times as fast as the base rhythm. Simply put, slow is about half the regular rhythm, fast is one and half times faster than the regular rhythm.

During the playing process, you will likely intuitively play anyway within this rhythm range. There will be times, however, where the rhythm may become very fast when building to a crescendo or very slow when ending a sequence or session. Again, tune in to the energy that is created as you move within and occasionally outside of the standard rhythm range.

Soft and Loud

The volume at which the gong is played depends upon how skillfully the gong player can tune in to the needs of the client. The gong produces a powerful sound regardless of the volume it is played. A softly played gong can create amazing changes in the client during a therapy session, even if not played too skillfully. A gong played loudly and badly, however, can be very harmful.

If you are a beginning gong player, or uncertain of your abilities, play softly. If you are afraid to play loudly, then please do not. Inexperienced players sometimes make the mistake of playing loudly because they have experienced the transformational effects of hearing an experienced player play in such a manner.

On the other hand, if you are confident in your abilities and have a wide range of experience in playing the gong in different situations, and your client also has experience with the gong played at louder volumes, then please use the powerful sound of the gong to its best effects by increasing the volume to its upper range. For certain clients, the gong can be played at its highest level, almost to the decibel level of white noise, for short periods in order to break up deep patterns, remove traumatic blocks, and release karmic tendencies, or samskaras, from past lives.

Regardless if you are playing softly or loudly, however, varying the range of the volume is an important component of gong therapy. Increasing the volume can create a climatic release in the client while decreasing the volume invites acceptance and relaxation. By moving the volume from soft to loud, and back again, an adjustment and integration can be made between the sympathetic nervous system (activated by the loud volume) and the parasympathetic nervous system (activated by the soft volume). This ability to shift the nervous system back and forth by varying the volume level can create a state of deep relaxation.

In general, a louder volume creates focus and expectation in the client while the softer volume allows for openness and acceptance. The gong therapist can thus use variation in the volume levels to good therapeutic effects.

Patterns and Contrasts: The Essence of Playing the Gong

The human mind creates an experience of the environment through contrasts: Is it cool or warm? Is it light or dark? Loud or quiet? It is only through the contrast of polarities that the mind can experience variations in the environment and notice the shift in perception.

Similarly, the mind works to create recognizable patterns and to identify recurring themes as it categorizes and builds ways of understanding itself and the outer environment.

This continual organization and re-organization of our inner and outer reality is based upon the ability to recognize patterns and then learn by contrasting the polarities that compose them. In art for example, a pattern of recognition is established through composition and then contrasted through various tones, colors and shades.

For example, a surrealistic painting by an artist like Salvador Dali when viewed for the first time challenges our previous way of patterning, or recognizing, a painting due to its radical new way of contrasting various elements. At that moment that the pattern is "broken," we are forced to re-create a new sense of the outer reality that is being presented to us. Similarly, a person who has only heard classical music performed undergoes a complete musical re-patterning when they hear jazz for the first time.

In the same way, the gong also challenges our sense of self and our inner reality when the gong player skillfully weaves into a pattern a multiplicity of tones and contrasts that inverts the mind and forces a reorganization of how we experience sound and sound patterns.

Consequently, playing the gong requires an ability to create therapeutic patterns of mallet strikes that are contrasted by varying the rhythm and the volume. It is the playing pattern that holds the mind and it is the contrasts that causes the mind to change and thus therapeutically transform.

Let's look at an example of therapeutic playing that demonstrates patterns and contrasts that vary over five phases of playing:

The Therapeutic Heart Beat

1) Playing Pattern and Baseline

Upward strike ↑ above the center of the gong
Downward strike ↓ below the center of the gong
Slow Rhythm ↓ Low Volume ↓

2) Playing Pattern and First Phase

Upward strike ↑ above the center of the gong
Downward strike ↓ below the center of the gong
Slow Rhythm ↓ Higher Volume ↑

3) Playing Pattern and Second Phase

Upward strike ↑ above the center of the gong
Upward strike ↑ above the center of the gong
Downward strike ↓ below the center of the gong
Faster Rhythm ↑ Same Volume ←→

4) Playing Pattern and Third Phase

Upward strike ↑ above the center of the gong
Upward strike ↑ above the center of the gong
Downward strike ↓ below the center of the gong
Downward strike ↓ below the center of the gong
Faster Rhythm ↑ Higher Volume ↑

5) Playing Pattern and Final Phase

Upward strike ↑ above the center of the gong
Downward strike ↓ below the center of the gong
Slower Rhythm ↓ Lower Volume ↓

Notice that the areas are consistent where the gong is struck (above the center and below the center) in order to create a pattern, and the variations in rhythm and volume serve as the contrasts within the pattern. The player can also vary the areas that the gong is struck as the contrast yet keep the volume and/or the rhythm the same to create the pattern.

In effect, the gong player creates patterns by holding one or two of the playing components constant (playing area, rhythm, or volume) while varying one or two of the other components for the contrast.

During a gong playing session a player may intuit multiple playing patterns, varying the areas of the gong that are struck as well as the rhythm and the volume in which they are played. Some patterns may be created in the moment that they are played while others are drawn from the player's previous experiences.

The various patterns, and the contrasts used within each pattern, are then sequenced through transitions which in turn contrast and build upon the previous pattern. A transition may be something as simple as a pause or silence in the playing process to indicate a change is taking place, or it can be a return to a previous playing pattern that signals to the listener the start of another cycle.

All of these patterns and transitions come naturally as the gong therapist achieves a connection between their energy, the client's energy and the responsiveness of the gong itself.

Until there is an ease and naturalness in this connection, the gong player can investigate and use the various therapeutic patterns outlined in this chapter.

Therapeutic Playing Patterns: Fundamental Examples

Theoretically there is an infinite amount of playing patterns available to the gong player. Typically, a playing pattern area consists of striking different areas of the gong in a repeated sequence. For most people, it will be increasingly difficult to discern a pattern once the player has exceeded twelve playing areas, and most playing pattern patterns typically consist of only two to six areas.

To more easily describe these basic playing patterns, the gong area will be designated by 14 percussion points on its surface as shown here:

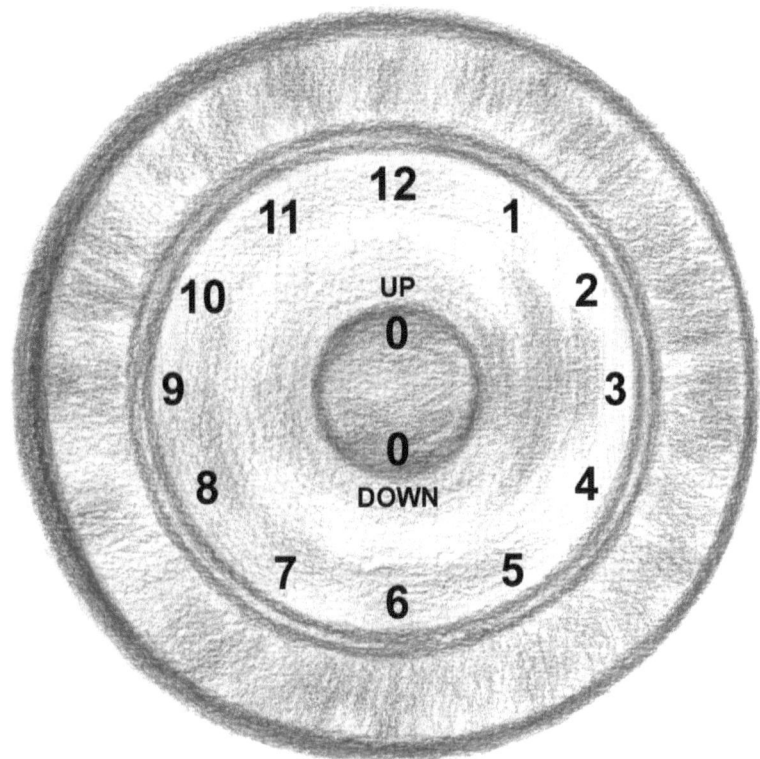

Using the percussion points, we can create an expression such as:

7 ➔ 5 ➔ 2

This indicates that the playing pattern is to strike the "7" percussion point, followed by the "5" percussion point and then the "2" percussion point. This playing sequence would then be repeated, with the rhythm and volume controlled and perhaps contrasted by the player.

The direction of the mallet strike on a point can also be indicated as up or down, such as an upward strike on the "2" percussion point (2↑) or a downward strike on the "7" percussion point 7↓.

The Heartbeat Pattern

This pattern was used in an earlier example:

0↑ → 0↓

repeating

This pattern is simple but effective in calming and centering the client when the sound and rhythm of a heartbeat are simulated.

The pattern can be altered to further simulate the natural sound of a heartbeat with three distinctive beats such as:

0↑ → 0↓ → 0↓

repeating

This basic therapeutic pattern is powerful in that by increasing the rhythm and volume you create a simulating effect or by slowing and quieting the rhythm and volume in contrast you can create a relaxing effect.

This is a good pattern to return to during a therapy session to re-center and re-set the client for patterns that may follow.

Polarity Patterns

These patterns are useful to create contrasting polarities in the energy of the client, and can be used to balance the right and left hemispheres of the brain and the two polarities of the client (male/female, projective/receptive, solar/lunar, etc.) in order to achieve an integration of self and resolve inner conflicts.

It is accomplished by playing the four diagonal percussion points of the gong (2, 8, 4 and 10) in one of several patterns:

Increases projection

8↓ →2↑ →8↓ →2↑

repeating

Increases reception

10↑ →4↓ →10↑ →4↓

repeating

Creates integration

8↓ →2↑ →10↑ →4↓ →8↓ →2↑ →10↑ →4↓

repeating

Balancing Patterns

These patterns are useful to return to during a gong therapy session as they balance and distribute the energies throughout the body.

The first balancing pattern releases and moves excessive energy or tension from the body in a clock-wise playing fashion:

$$3 \rightarrow 6 \rightarrow 9 \rightarrow 12 \rightarrow 3 \rightarrow 6 \rightarrow 9 \rightarrow 12$$

repeating

The second balancing pattern builds and activates energy in the body in a counter clock-wise playing fashion:

$$9 \rightarrow 12 \rightarrow 3 \rightarrow 6 \rightarrow 9 \rightarrow 12 \rightarrow 3 \rightarrow 6$$

repeating

These two patterns can be alternated to release blocked energy, particularly if the rhythms and volumes are contrasted during the playing:

$$3 \rightarrow 6 \rightarrow 9 \rightarrow 12 \rightarrow 3 \rightarrow 6 \rightarrow 9 \rightarrow 12$$
$$9 \rightarrow 12 \rightarrow 3 \rightarrow 6 \rightarrow 9 \rightarrow 12 \rightarrow 3 \rightarrow 6$$

repeating

Another balancing pattern that works to activate or sedate the energy centers or chakras of the body is to play the gong from bottom to top (activate) or top to bottom (sedate) as follows.

Elevation and moving energy to the upper chakras:

$$6\downarrow \rightarrow 0\downarrow \rightarrow 0\uparrow \rightarrow 12\uparrow$$

repeating

Grounding and moving energy to the lower chakras:

$$12\uparrow \rightarrow 0\uparrow \rightarrow 0\downarrow \rightarrow 6\downarrow$$

repeating

These two patterns can be alternated to release blocked energy in the chakras, particularly if the rhythm and volume is increased in the first pattern and decreases during the second pattern are contrasted during the playing:

$$6\uparrow \rightarrow 0\uparrow \rightarrow 0\uparrow \rightarrow 12\uparrow$$
$$12\downarrow \rightarrow 0\downarrow \rightarrow 0\downarrow \rightarrow 6\downarrow$$

repeating

Hypnotic Monotones

A simple pattern for inducing self-hypnosis and suspended thoughts is a steady rhythmical beat on one area of the gong with a variation in the volume. There are several effective percussion points to produce these hypnotic monotones, including points 11, 12 or 1 and points or 5, 6 or 7. The mallet is held at one of these points, near the surface, while continuously tapping the point in a continuous and moderately slow rhythm, allowing the volume to slightly increase and then subside, almost like the waves of the ocean that break and then return to the sea.

This pattern can be continued for 1 to 3 minutes to entrance the listener into a non-judgmental state before playing more complex patterns. For this reason, this playing technique is sometimes used at the beginning of a therapy session.

Binaural Beats

The gong is adept at producing what are termed binaural beats, or binaural tones, by simultaneously creating one sound of two different frequencies that are heard by the listener as one tone. When this occurs, brainwave frequencies begin to align with the tones to create a state of brainwave entrainment that leads to an open susceptibility to sound patterns that may follow.

To practice creating binaural beats with the gongs, two mallets of different sizes are struck slightly out of sync in a repeated pattern to create a pulsing sound. Ideally there is only a small offset in the frequencies of the two tones created by the two mallets. This beat can also be approximated with only one mallet, by quickly striking two areas slightly off-center so that the two tones blend into one sound.

Any two percussion points on the gong may be used, and they are repeated struck in much in the same way as the hypnotic monotones.

The Two Healing Polarities: Langhana and Brimhana

A traditional way to promote healing and transformation through gong therapy is by using the two healing approaches described in the Vedic science of Ayurveda that categorizes all therapies as being essentially either *Brimhana* (expansion) or *Langhana* (reduction) in nature.

Therapeutic practices, according the ancient healing science of Ayurveda, that promote *brimhana* increase vitality and build energy in the body while therapies that foster *langhana* are grounding and calming.

In summary, these are the qualities associated with these two healing polarities:

Langhana Qualities	Brimhana Qualities
Cooling	Warming
Relaxing	Activating
Release energy	Build energy
Promote elimination	Promote strengthening
Aid parasympathetic nervous system	Aid sympathetic nervous system
Increase sensory activity	Increase motor activity

Therapeutic **Langhana** practices are used to treat these types of illnesses:

- Tension
- Stress
- Insomnia
- Constipation
- Headaches
- Chronic pain
- Irritability
- Arthritis
- Stroke
- Allergies
- Inflammation

Therapeutic **Brimhana** practices are used to treat these types of illnesses:

- Fatigue
- Low Vitality
- Lethargy
- Diarrhea
- Poor Circulation
- Depression
- Asthma
- Chronic Fatigue
- Apathy
- Weakness

For example, an Ayurvedic practitioner might use herbs that have Brimhana qualities (such as ginger) to increase circulation or cooling foods that encourage Langhana (such as aloe vera) to reduce inflammation. In a similar way, the gong therapist can also play the gong in different ways to bring either the qualities of Brimhana or Langhana into the therapy session.

Playing the Gong for Langhana and Brimhana

The gong player creates either a Langhana or Brimhana effect by controlling the rhythm, modulating the volume, and by striking different playing areas of the gong. The general guidelines for playing techniques to create a Langhana or Brimhana effect are as follows:

Playing Rhythm

Langhana ← Slower Rhythm   Faster Rhythm → Brimhana

Playing Volume

Langhana ← Softer Volume   Louder Volume → Brimhana

Gong Playing Areas

Langhana ← Bottom Half   Top Half → Brimhana

Mallet Strikes

Langhana ← Downward Strike   Upward Strike → Brimhana

Remember that Langhana contracts and sedates while Brimhana expands and activates. While one of these effects may be the dominant experience during a gong therapy session depending upon the condition that is being addressed, the therapist should also use these two approaches in balance and contrast.

Practicing the therapeutic playing techniques described in this chapter is an excellent way for the beginning and intermediate gong player to discover and refine new ways of playing for a gong therapy session. Yet ultimately they are only an entry point for your own journey of self-discovery as you play. While techniques and the gongs themselves allow for the expression of gong therapy, it is always the gong player's intuition and their spiritual practice that allow the healing effects promised by this modality to be delivered.

As the tone of the individual being is one and many, so the tone of a gong is one and many.

Touch it lightly at the center, then farther, farther away until you reach the outer edge.

You hear an infinite gradation of sub-tones all of which concur to form the compound tone of the gong.

Each tone an individual being yet all bound in a perfect metallic solidarity, all blending their voices into the great tone-entity, heard when the center is struck. In that single tone you have a complete organic symphony.

Such a tone is the beginning and end of music, the seed of all music.

Dane Rudhyar

Group Gong Therapy

There may be opportunities to offer gong therapy sessions for several people at a time rather than for an individual. Examples are a session for a support group to help them with a specific condition, or to introduce interested clients to the benefits of gong therapy or as part of a yoga class or other group mind-body practice.

A group therapy session does require different approaches in the assessment process, the therapy environment, and the methodology than is used in a one-on-one session.

Group Assessment

Since the gongs are played for a group rather than for an individual, the therapist needs to determine a group intention for the session rather than a personal assessment. For example, if there is a shared commonality of the group, such as people who are in addiction recovery or who have a specific physical (cancer survivors, pain management, etc.) or emotional (depression, anger, grief, etc.) condition, the therapy session can be structured to address that issue.

On the other hand, if it is a mixed group, then the therapist needs to self-select a suitable positive intention for the healing that is to occur, such as a session to release fear, develop self-compassion, strengthen the immune system, and so on.

For example, group therapy sessions may focus on balancing the chakras, reducing stress, or simply being better prepared to deal with the group's shared experience, such as a change in seasons or a challenging work environment.

Consideration needs to be given to the range of differences in the group, such as age, physical capability, and previous experience with yoga, sound healing or alternative healing approaches.

Group Therapy Environment

In a group session, the clients will ideally be able to relax on their backs with suitable support. In some environments (such as an office or school classroom), it will be necessary to have the group sit in chairs or on the floor.

The placement and selection of the gongs may be different for a group session. The gongs are placed some distance from the clients rather than the close-in arrangement for a private session. If there is more than one gong available, they may need to be spaced around the room to create a more enclosed experience of the sound (and in this case, there may be more than one gong player).

The gongs for a group can be larger than normally used in a private session, the 32 to 38 inch (80 to 100 cm) size gongs are recommended if available. Another excellent option is to use smaller gongs that can be held by hand and played while moving around the group during the session, again taking care that the hand-held gongs do not create anxiety by overly close proximity to individuals.

Group Therapy Methodology

Because you will not be able to individually instruct people, you may wish to select a simple or single methodology to support the gong playing session. For example, a hand position or mudra that can be easily held is ideal and can be selected to enhance the intention for the group session.

Given that there is not the intimacy between therapist and client that exists in a private therapy session, a group therapy session is generally more successful when attention is given to creating a group energy or consciousness as part of the preparation for the actual gong playing.

This group energy can be accomplished by several means: meditation, chanting, prayer, ritual, yoga practice, exercise, or dance. You can also accomplish a feeling of group consciousness by arranging the participants in a circle and allowing them to share why they are here or what their intention for the healing session. In such an arrangement, the gongs can then be played inside or around the circle.

Group Therapy Yoga Classes

An excellent way to create a group consciousness and receptivity for the therapy session is to practice a yoga class that incorporates the sound of the gong within the class. Many yoga classes can easily be adapted into Gong Yoga classes (*Teaching Gong Yoga*), and Kundalini Yoga classes are excellent preparation for group gong therapy sessions.

Here are two Kundalini yoga practices specifically given by Yogi Bhajan for gong therapy.

Gong Therapy: Releasing Fear

This gong therapy session given by Yogi Bhajan uses a pranayama technique called Breath of Fire. The breath is panted through the nose with the mouth closed, equal inhale and equal exhale, from 1 to 2 times per second. The breath is light and easy, lifted into the heart, without pumping the belly. If you are unfamiliar with this technique, please consult a Kundalini Yoga teacher.

This session allows for the release of deep subconscious fears that limit our sense of self. It is important to relax and "float" with the sound of the gong and to relax for 10 minutes after the gong playing ends.

This practice and the one following it uses a Kundalini Yoga breathing practice called Breath of Fire. The breath is distinguished by a quick and equal active inhale and active exhale through the nose as if lightly panting with the mouth closed. There is an equal intensity and length of the inhale and the exhale, at the rate of 1 to 3 breaths per second. The heart is lifted and the solar plexus lightly dances with the breath, yet the movement is not forceful or contractive. The breath is rhythmical (equal length between inhale and exhale) and quick (1 to 3 breaths per second) so a continuous light panting breath through the nose is accomplished without strain.

How to Do It:

- Come sitting on the heels. Use a blanket between the calves and thighs if you need the support.

- Raise the arms over the head, the elbows are straight yet the shoulders are relaxed and not pulled up around the neck. The palms are place flat together with the fingers and thumbs of both hands pressed together and pointing upward.

- Long deep breathing for one minute.

- Inhale, and begin the Breath of Fire while the gong is played for one minute. Stop playing the gong.

- Inhale, keep the arms up and hands with long deep breathing for one minute while the sound of the gong fades away.

- Inhale, and begin the Breath of Fire as the gong is played at a faster rhythm and louder volume for one minute. Stop playing.

- Inhale, keep the arms up and hands with long deep breathing for one minute while the sound of the gong fades away.

- Inhale, and begin the Breath of Fire as the gong is played at a faster rhythm and louder volume for one minute. Stop playing.

- Inhale, keep the arms up and hands with long deep breathing for one minute or until the sound of the gong fades away completely. Exhale completely. Inhale deeply.

- Retain the breath and pull the energy up the spine.

- Exhale and deeply relax on the back.

Gong Therapy: Nervous System Regeneration

This gong therapy session was originally given by Yogi Bhajan to use in a rehabilitation program to regenerate the nervous systems of drug users. For group therapy sessions, it is also highly effective to ameliorate the deleterious effects of chronic stress.

How to Do It:
- Sit in a comfortable upright posture. Breathe in through the left nostril and out through the right nostril by using the thumb of the right hand to block the right nostril when you inhale through the left nostril and one of the fingers to block the left nostril as you exhale through the right nostril. Continue to inhale left and exhale right for 5 to 10 minutes. Then inhale deeply and direct the closed eyes upward to the brow point (third eye). Retain the breath for as long as comfortable.

- Now reverse the breath pattern. Breathe in through the right nostril and out through the left nostril. Continue to inhale right and exhale left for 5 to 10 minutes. Then inhale deeply and direct the closed eyes upward to the brow point (third eye). Retain the breath for as long as comfortable.

- Press the palms together at the center of the chest with the fingers pointing up. Begin the Breath of Fire (see description of this breath in the previous section). Continue for 3 to 5 minutes. Then inhale, and exhale completely. Hold the breath out for 10-20 seconds as you press the palms firmly together. Inhale and then exhale.

- Continue sitting. Touch the thumb tip to the tip of the index finger of both hands and then relax the hand position over the knees. The eyes are held 1/10 open. Curl the tongue into a "U" shape and extend the tip past the lips. Inhale deeply over the tongue. Close the mouth, exhale through the nose. Continue for 3 to 5 minutes. Then inhale deeply, and retain the breath for 15 to 60 seconds. Exhale through the nose.

- Remain sitting. Relax the left hand palm up in the lap. Rest the back of the right hand in the left palm. Touch the thumb tips together. Focus the eyes past the tip of the nose. Inhale in four equal segments with a slight pause after each segment:

- Inhale $1/4^{th}$ of the breath. Inhale the second $1/4^{th}$ of breath. Inhale the third $1/4^{th}$ of breath. Finally inhale the last $1/4^{th}$ of breath. As you inhale, mentally repeat SA (on first segment), TA (on second), NA (on third), MA (on last segment).

- Exhale powerfully in one long stroke through the nose. As you exhale, mentally repeat the mantra WHA-HEY GUROO.

- Continue the four-part inhale and one-part exhale with the silent sounds for 5 to 11 minutes. Then inhale deeply and hold briefly as you roll the eyes upward.

- Relax for the gong playing session. Interlace the fingers of the hands and rest them over the navel point. Actively listen to the sound of the gong and let yourself freely travel into the sound.

Begin to Play the Gong

- Play a steady rhythm and medium volume around the center of the gong, striking upward downward above the center and below the center, as if loose brushing the mallet back and forth. Play this way 3 to 5 minutes

- Switch to a continuous and blended tone, playing the diagonal percussion points 8 and 12 for a while and then striking the up 0 and down 0 points back and forth. Move between these two patterns. Play this way 3 to 5 minutes.

- Switch to playing the gong along the outer rim to create a light swishing sound. Play this way 3 to 5 minutes.

- Repeat these three patterns 3 to 5 times for a total of 45 minutes playing time.

Relax deeply for 10 minutes. Come out of the relaxation and take 5 to 10 deep breaths. Then drink two glasses of water.

Gong is the sound

That projects you out of your realm

To the Infinity.

Yogi Bhajan

Gong Therapy as a Profession

Gong Therapy in the early twenty-first century is still in its infancy, both as a healing practice and as a recognized profession. Few books have been written on the gong, and we are the first generation of Western gong healers. Yet, it is not immature nor without its precedents. In various ways, sound healers, yogis and shamans have practiced this healing modality for hundreds of years.

What is new is that the gong itself is now available to many people, and not just the select few, and is being embraced by professionals in both traditional and alternative healing professions.

While there is no recognized occupation as a gong therapist, no widely accepted standards for training or certification, and only nascent research to validate its effectiveness, Gong Therapy does live in the hands of yoga teachers and sound healers. And despite that these two professions are only beginning to find acceptance in the dominant healthcare paradigm, there is a sense of momentum as more people experience the sound of the gong. Its immediate and easy accessibility, and its universal language – sound – bring unexpected healing in the moment it is delivered.

We who have practiced and experienced Gong Therapy know it works, much in the same way that Westerners who experienced such formerly esoteric healing practices as Ayurveda and acupuncture know that they too give results.

Like other emergent healing modalities, Gong Therapy will first be nurtured as an adjunct profession, not wholly able to be stand by itself but more and more widely employed by sound healers, yoga teachers, massage therapists, nurses, energy workers, music therapists, psychotherapists and alternative healers in their own healing and therapy work.

Gong Therapy Today

The applications for Gong Therapy as part of the alternative and complementary healthcare field are limitless. The gong has always been used to mark and ease life transitions, so we are seeing its use by midwives before and during the birthing process and by hospice nurses for end of life patients.

The gong has been used since the early 1970s for treatment of addictions and for those in recovery programs. Psychotherapists are reporting beneficial results for patients who suffer from depression, anxiety and even anger. In Sweden the gong is now part of a medical yoga program, and in Greece there has been growing interest and acceptance of its use in the nursing profession.

Children with special needs, disadvantaged youth, and students with learning disabilities have responded favorably to it use in the classroom as well.

While it may not be a widely recognized independent profession, it has been subsumed into many professions already, to be used first as an adjunct modality and eventually as an important component.

Gong Therapy Tomorrow

The gong, and gong therapy, will be widely accepted in Western culture within twenty years, even surpassing the yoga revolution of the late twentieth century because its potential audience is unlimited and its entry requirements are non-existent. Simply relax and listen.

In the latter half of this century, gong temples will be commonplace, and gong treatments at the end of the day will be the normal way to recharge and relax. Those who facilitate and develop gong therapy today will be the keepers and practitioners of this healing art tomorrow. It will be more than a profession – it will be a sacred calling and a spiritual endeavor that will change the world because the sound of the gong is the source of all creation and all healing. Until then –

Play the Gong. Heal the World. Peace, Love and Sat Nam.

God created the Universe

With this sound of the gong.

Fly with it,

Spread your wings and go with it,

Flow away.

Yogi Bhajan

About the Author

Mehtab Benton is originator of Gong Yoga™ and author of *Gong Yoga: Healing and Enlightenment Through Sound,* published in five international editions and translations. His book *Teaching Gong Yoga* is the first book on using yoga practices with the gong, and his DVD course *How to Play the Gong* is a best-selling video for beginning and intermediate players. His latest book, *Gong Therapy*, has been used in courses around the world by yoga teachers, sound healers, and therapists.

A practitioner and teacher of Kundalini Yoga for over 40 years, Mehtab has trained hundreds of teachers. He is a certified Vedic Astrologer, a mentor in the American College of Vedic Astrology, and author of Astrology Yoga, the first comprehensive book on using the science of Jyotish in the practice and teaching of yoga. Mehtab has an educational background in psychology and yoga therapy and the author of 15 books.

He conducts workshops and trainings in Gong Yoga and Gong Therapy internationally.

**He may be contacted through his website:
www.gongteacher.com**

Teaching Gong Yoga

Theory & Practice

Mehtab Benton

Teaching Gong Yoga is the first comprehensive book on using the sound of the Gong to enhance the practices of Yoga, including asana, pranayama, mantra, meditation and relaxation.

Gong players, sound healers, yoga teachers, and students will learn how the gong can be used in all types of yoga, including:

**Kundalini Yoga • Hatha Yoga • Vinyasa Flow Yoga • Ashtanga Yoga
Restorative Yoga • Prenatal Yoga • Children's Yoga • Senior's Yoga**

You will learn the theory and practice for:

- Constructing and teaching Gong Yoga classes
- Playing the Gong for the chakras
- Practicing meditation with the Gong
- Using gong maps to develop your playing techniques
- Creating deep relaxation and healing through the Gong

Fully illustrated with nearly 100 drawings and 23 tables of information on these and other topics:

**Asana Sequences with the Gong
Sound, Prana and the Five Tattvas
Playing the Gong for the Chakras
Pranayama Practices and the Gong
The Gong, Mantras and the Inner Sounds
Mudras and Gong Meditation
The Gong and Yoga Nidra
PLUS special yoga practices for gong players and teachers**

www.gongteacher.com

Gong Yoga

Healing and Enlightenment Through Sound

Mehtab Benton

Gong Yoga is the first comprehensive book on practicing and teaching yoga with the sound of the gong. You will learn about the origin, history and use of the gong for yoga and meditation as well as its current therapeutic applications for healing and transformation.

The book contains a step-by-step training guide to teach you how to play the gong through a series of practice sessions. You will learn the basic techniques to play the gong as well as advanced techniques to create your own gong playing sessions. You will learn how to structure gong yoga classes and gong yoga therapy sessions for your students and clients.

A comprehensive chapter on Yoga and the Gong describes the chakras, the major energy channels of the body (the nadis), and the five sheaths of existence (the koshas), that are key to understanding how the gong integrates with the practice of yoga. Special sections explain the use of Kundalini Yoga mantras for playing the gong, how to select and care for your gong and additional resources to develop your skills.

Written by a long-time yoga teacher and international trainer of students and therapists in the art of playing the gong for meditation and healing.

*"Information on how to play the gong and the spiritual aspects of the sound of the gong are difficult to find. **GONG YOGA** is a wonderful introduction to all aspects of the gong and the yoga that is associated with it. The interesting history of the gong, its uses in Western and Eastern music, how to play it and the gong's effects on the body's energetic system are all discussed. FIVE STARS!"*

www.gongteacher.com

How to Play the Gong

DVD Training Course

Mehtab Benton

How to Play the Gong is the complete video instructional course for self-study and mastery of the gong.

Performed and written by Mehtab Benton, author of GONG YOGA, this two-volume DVD course demonstrates both basic and advanced playing techniques through a series of practice sessions.

Volume 1 introduces you to the different playing areas of the gong, specific percussion points, and working with the mallet strikes to control volume and create rhythms.

Volume 2 begins with using combination strokes to create a rich wall of sound and then building into more intricate sequences. You'll learn how to use multiple mallets and several gongs to create an extended sound session through intuitive playing. *Bonus features* include using the gong with the chakras and a live outdoor performance.

Playing the gong does not require any prior musical experience. You begin with the basic mallet strokes, learn playing sequences and then create your own gong sessions for relaxation, meditation, and healing.

Mehtab Benton is the author of *Gong Yoga: Healing and Enlightenment Through Sound*, and the master teacher of the video course *How to Play the Gong*. He has trained hundreds of yoga teachers and therapists in the art and science of playing the gong. He is an Integrative Yoga Therapist and yoga teacher trainer with a background in counseling and psychology.

www.gongteacher.com

Astrology Yoga

Cosmic Cycles of Transformation

Mehtab Benton

Astrology Yoga is the first comprehensive book on the practice of Yoga using the ancient science of Vedic Astrology, or Jyotish.

Written for yoga practitioners with a limited knowledge of astrology, this book explains the dynamic and vital relationship that has always existed between these two ancient Vedic sciences and how you can use this knowledge to accelerate your transformation by working with your personal planetary energies.

You will learn about your yogic Sun sign and Moon sign, the specific karmic issues in your life, the most appropriate yoga practices based on your birth date, and the most beneficial times to do your yoga practices over the day, during the week, and throughout all the cycles of your life.

The book describes the original relationship between Eastern or Vedic astrology and yoga and the differences between Yoga astrology and western astrology. You'll learn about the nine major planetary energies, the twelve signs, and the twelve life areas of astrology yoga.

You will learn about your own astrological life cycles that affect your consciousness and yoga practices, as well as the universal cosmic cycles that affect everyone. Yoga practices for moon phases, days of the week, months of the year, and hours of the day, as well as for special occasions of the solstices, equinoxes and eclipses, are discussed to help you design a yoga practice that supports you through each cycle of your life.

Written by a life-long practitioner and teacher of Yoga as well as a certified Vedic astrologer, Astrology Yoga provides you with a personal roadmap for your journey to enlightenment.

www.astrologyteacher.com

About Bookshelf Press

Bookshelf Press is a print and electronic publisher of books on yoga, health, Eastern astrology, and the art and science of playing the gong.

Rights are available through the publisher for foreign editions and other media adaptations.

Wholesale and retail orders are available directly from the publisher.

www.bookshelfpress.com

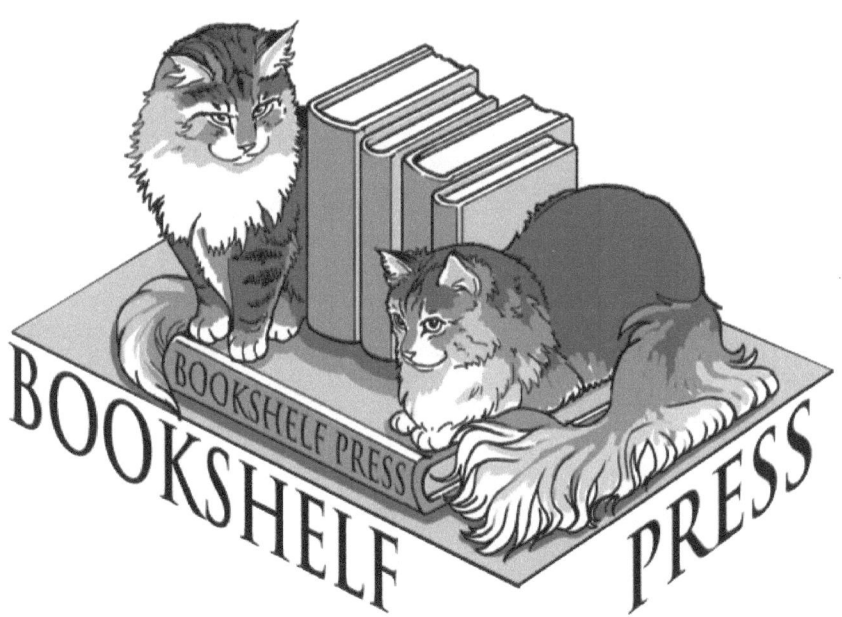

www.ingramcontent.com/pod-product-compliance
Lightning Source LLC
LaVergne TN
LVHW092007090526
838202LV00001B/37